CURLS,
CURLS,
CURLS!

Your Go-To Guide for Rocking Curly Hair — Plus Tutorials for 60 Fabulous Looks

---

SAMANTHA HARRIS

CHRONICLE BOOKS
SAN FRANCISCO

First published in the United States of America in 2016 by Chronicle Books LLC.

Library of Congress Cataloging-in-Publication Data available.

ISBN: 978-1-4521-5834-1

Manufactured in China.

Publisher: Mark Searle
Editorial Director: Isheeta Mustafi
Commissioning Editor: Alison Morris
Editor: Angela Koo
Junior Editor: Abbie Sharman
Art Director: Michelle Rowlandson
Book layout: Agata Rybicka and Richard Peters
Illustrations: Sarah Skeate
Photography: Yolanda Diaz

10 9 8 7 6 5 4 3 2 1

Chronicle Books LLC
680 Second Street
San Francisco, CA 94107
www.chroniclebooks.com

Image credits
Front cover: Hair Samantha Harris; photography Yolanda Diaz; models (clockwise from top) Aly Hill, Nicole Baulknight, and Cage Cluff.

Back cover: Hair Samantha Harris; photography Yolanda Diaz; models (top to bottom) Tiffany Marie Stephens, Bethany Shedrick, and Rachel Jordan.

This book is dedicated to my nephews and nieces: Joshua, Jordan, Faith, and Journey. May all your dreams come true.

CONTENTS

▶ BUNS AND KNOTS

▶ BRAIDS AND TWISTS

▶ RESOURCES

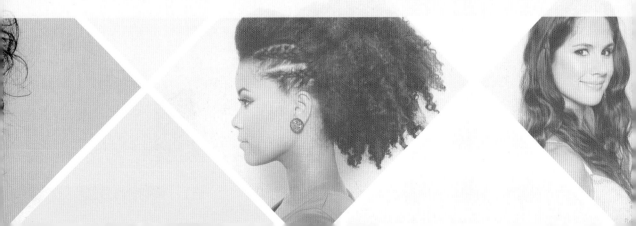

VISUAL INDEX

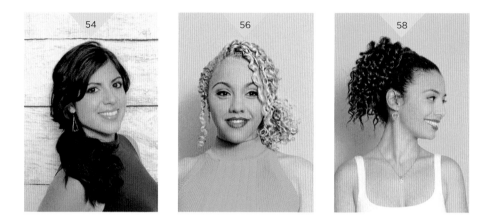

54

56

58

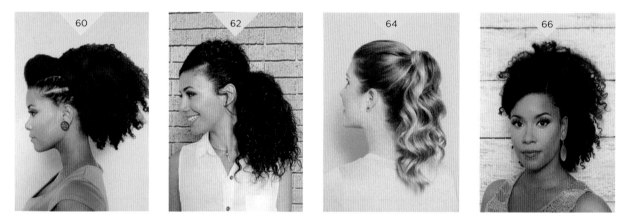

60

62

64

66

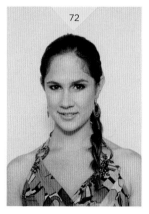
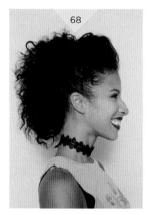
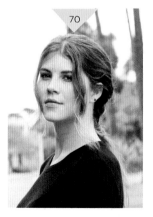

68

70

72

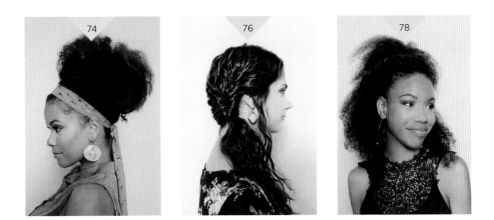

74

76

78

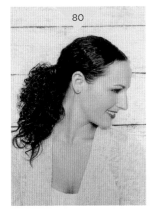

80

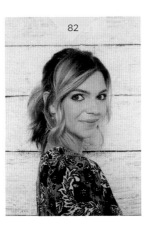

82

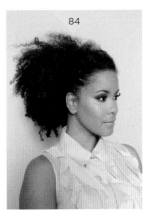

84

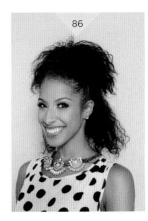

86

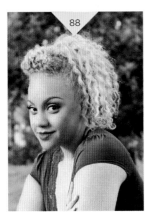

88

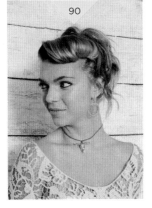

90

92

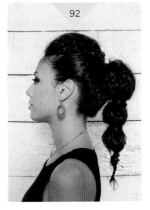

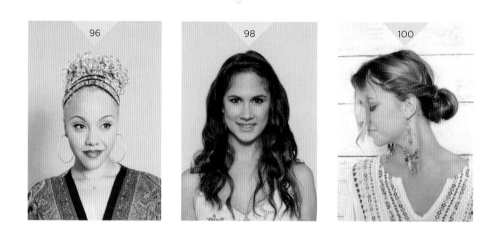

96   98   100

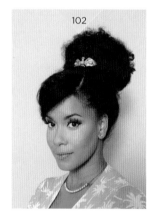

102

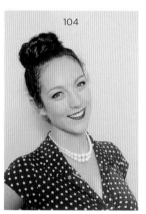

104

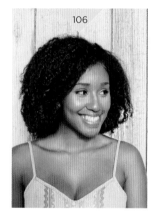

106

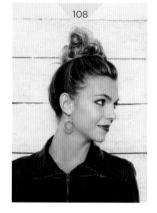

108

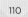

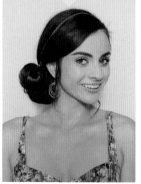

110

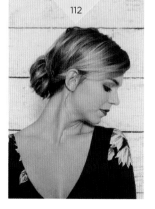

112

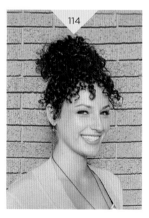

114

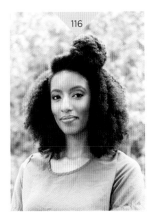

116

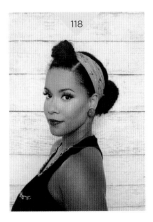

118

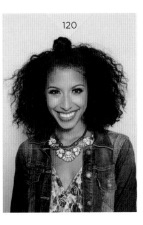

120

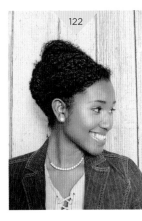

122

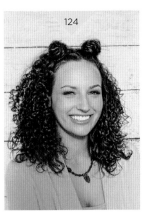

124

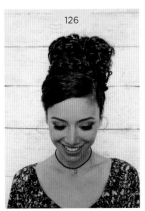

126

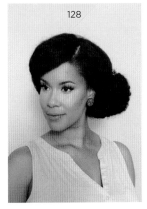

128

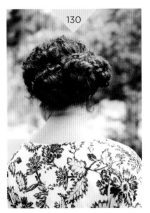

130

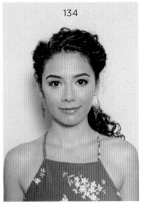

134

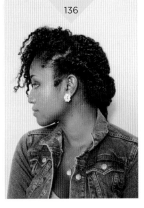

136

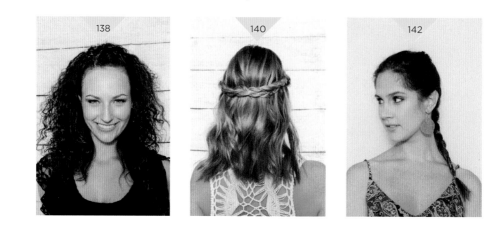

138 140 142

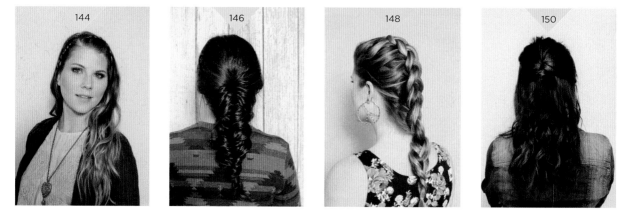

144 146 148 150

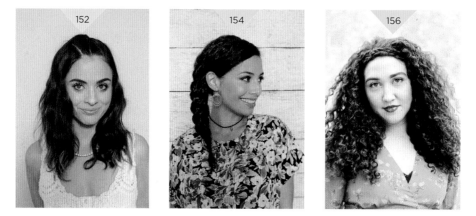

152 154 156

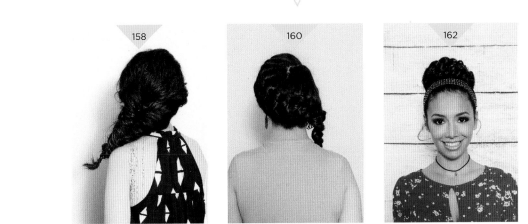

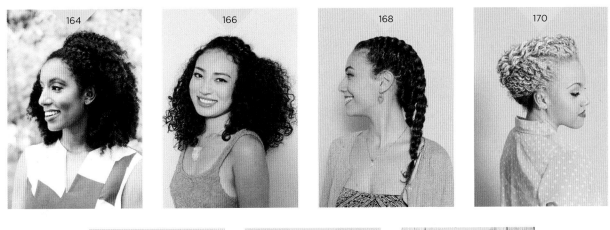

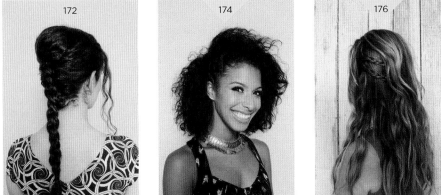

INTRODUCTION

Hi, I'm Samantha Harris. Online and in the natural-hair community I am known as Ahfro Baang, and for years I have shared my simple, "do-it-yourself" hairstyle tutorials as well as tips and tricks to care for curly hair. After suffering from relaxer damage, I chopped off most of my hair and started on a journey that consisted of learning how to understand and care for my natural curls. As I transitioned away from chemically straightened hair, I came to learn what worked and what didn't, which was an exciting experience! I also engaged with a community of curlies from all over the world, gathering lots of tips from them along the way.

Curly hair comes in lots of shapes and sizes, so the first step is figuring out your own curl type and how to keep it looking at its best every day. Choosing the right products is a must, so I've included summaries of nine different curl types with accompanying suggestions—just read through, identify your closest match, and work out a routine that works for you. You may find that a mix-and-match approach is the best solution. That's fine—just make sure you stick to it! I've also provided plenty of tips and tricks for permed and color-treated hair, as well as hair that is recovering from being chemically straightened, which—as I know—can require lots of extra TLC. And, if you have some time on your hands, why not try experimenting with some homemade remedies?

Too much heat is a bad thing for your hair, so I have included four easy tutorials for curling your hair without heat. These are suitable for curlies and non-curlies alike, so trying these out could be a great place to start.

I have then put together a set of 60 fabulous curly hairstyles, grouped in three categories for easy selection—Ponytails, Buns and Knots, and Braids and Twists. You'll find something to suit every occasion here. While hair is the main focus, I have also included makeup and accessory tips to help inspire you in the creation of a finished look. Each tutorial consists of five easy-to-follow steps, so just follow these closely and be sure to check the top tips for each one, and you will be on your way to achieving perfect results every time!

Samantha Harris

Samantha Harris

RIGHT: High bun with swooped bangs, page 102

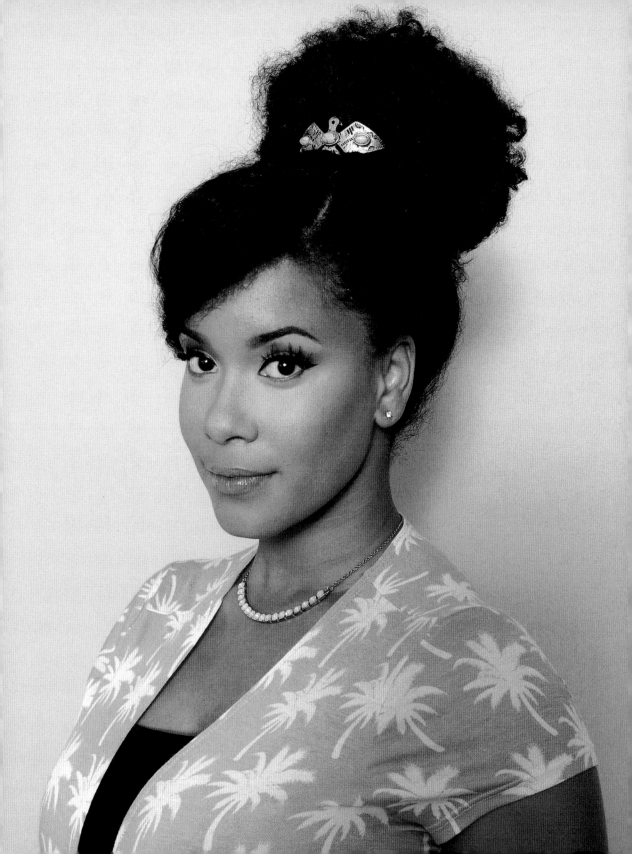

HAIR CARE

TYPES OF CURLY HAIR

IDENTIFYING YOUR CURL

If you have curly hair, then you probably already know that there is not just one type of curl out there. Learning how best to care for your hair, and how to make the most of it when styling, depends on knowing your own particular curl type.

To help you identify where you fall on the "curl spectrum," the following few pages break down curly hair into three overall categories—waves, curls, and coils. Each of these categories is then further subdivided, with each curl type being more curly than the last, to provide nine distinct curl types overall.

From the descriptions and accompanying photos you can pinpoint the closest match to your own hair. You may find that your curls share characteristics with more than one of these types, in which case just experiment with the suggestions offered here to come up with your own bespoke regimen!

CURLY WAVES

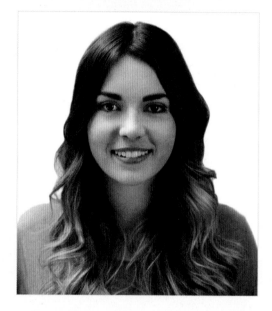

This curl type has the slightest curl pattern. Products penetrate the hair easily but too much moisture will weigh hair down. Use lightweight moisturizing products that provide adequate hold without any unwanted weight.

QUICK TIPS

• Avoid brushing your hair whenever possible, and detangle it using your fingers to avoid frizz.

• Use a diffuser and flip your head over while working at the roots to create more volume.

• Avoid heavy products that weigh down curls and clog hair follicles.

PERFECT PRODUCTS

• Gentle, sulfate-free, volumizing shampoos and conditioners

• Mousse or lightweight styling milk

• Water-based leave-in conditioner (for refreshing hair when needed)

• Avocado hair mask (see page 34)

BEACH WAVES

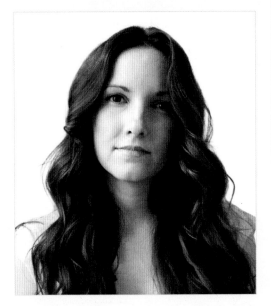

Beach waves are generally fine, have a tendency to lose definition, and can be prone to frizz. This hair type absorbs excess oils easily, so products that encourage moisture without weighing down your hair are best.

QUICK TIPS

• After applying your curl definer, flip your head over and use your fingers to gently scrunch the hair upward to encourage the natural curl pattern.

• Use a diffuser attachment when blow-drying to avoid creating frizz.

• Two-strand-twist your curls at night to increase the wave pattern (see the tutorial on pages 48–49).

PERFECT PRODUCTS
• Volumizing shampoos and conditioners

• Foaming mousse or light curl definer on wet hair

• Leave-in conditioner spray (for refreshing hair when needed)

TIGHT WAVES

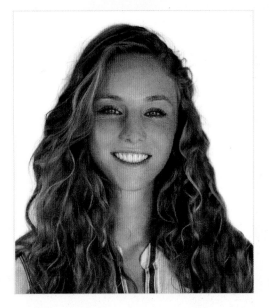

Tight waves have the most natural definition of all of the wave types. Although they can still lose definition easily, they are actually heavier and thicker than their less-coiled counterparts. If you have tight waves, you should look out for lightweight products that will combat frizz effectively but won't weigh down your hair.

QUICK TIPS

• When styling wet hair, divide your hair into four sections and then use your fingers to rake through any styling products for thorough distribution.

• After your styling product has been raked through, scrunch your hair from the ends back to the roots to promote a more defined curl.

PERFECT PRODUCTS
• Volumizing shampoos and conditioners

• Curl definer and styling milk

• Deep-conditioning and protein treatments

LOOSE CURLS

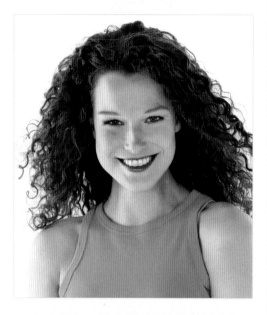

Loose curls have a springy, wide, S-shaped pattern, and the hair itself is a lot thicker and heavier than the tight waves on page 17. You will still need to stick to a lightweight moisturizing formula for your shampoo and conditioner, though, and use a definer to combat frizz.

QUICK TIPS

• For definition, use your fingers to rake products throughout your hair.

• After applying your styling product, finger-coil individual strands to enhance the definition.

• While blow-drying, flip your head over and lift it at the roots while you work for added volume.

PERFECT PRODUCTS

• Moisturizing shampoos and conditioners

• A mix of leave-in conditioner spray and styling milk for moisture and definition

• Protein treatments

SPIRAL CURLS

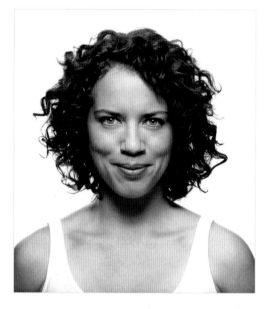

This curl type has more definition than the loose curl, and the S-shape is more prominent, although smaller in size. This type also has more volume than the other curl types. Because of its density, it does suffer from frizz and needs more emollient-rich products, which will seep through and moisturize each strand while providing definition.

QUICK TIPS

• Give yourself a scalp massage before washing, this increases blood flow which helps to maintain a healthy scalp and encourage strong growth.

• Use a diffuser when blow-drying to avoid frizz.

PERFECT PRODUCTS

• Sulfate-free moisturizing shampoos and conditioners.

• Silicone-free styling milk

• Clarifying shampoo once a month to deep-cleanse the hair

TIGHT CURLS

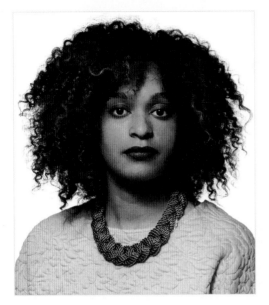

This corkscrew shape is smaller and thicker than the spiral. It is also more prone to dryness and frizz, so maintain a weekly moisturizing routine. Use a shampoo containing tea tree oil to combat dryness at the scalp, and apply moisturizing hair masks and deep conditioners one to two times a week. Seal the ends with coconut oil to retain moisture.

QUICK TIPS

• Use a hair steamer to open the hair cuticles and allow for better product absorption.
• Use the LOC method to seal the cuticles and retain moisture (see page 40).

PERFECT PRODUCTS

• Alternate between a sulfate-free shampoo and one containing tea tree oil
• Lotions, foaming mousse, and lightweight gel
• Deep conditioners and hair masks

LOOSE COILS

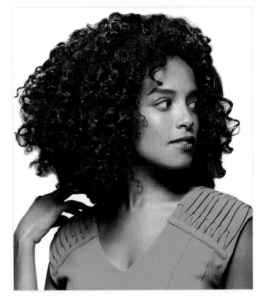

Loosely coiled hair still has a strong curl pattern, but it also has more of a Z-shape. This hair type is coarse, dense, and very prone to dryness, so choose products that will promote scalp health and clean the hair without stripping it of its natural oils. You should also select styling products that will help with moisture retention.

QUICK TIPS

• Use a steamer during any deep-conditioning session to open up the hair cuticles for better absorption.
• When styling, use oil as the final product to lock in moisture (see the LCO method, page 40).

PERFECT PRODUCTS

• Alternate between tea-tree-oil shampoo and moisturizing co-wash (see page 24)
• Deep-conditioning and oil treatments

SPIRAL COILS

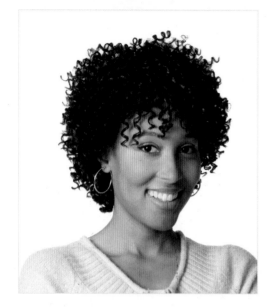

Spiral coils can be coarse. They have a wiry feel and the coils are densely packed together. This hair type also suffers from hair shrinkage and tends to have a lower porosity, which can make it harder to retain moisture. Since hair is left susceptible to breakage, stick to products that help with moisture retention.

QUICK TIPS

- Use the LCO or LOC method to retain moisture (see page 40).
- Use twist-outs to stretch hair to its actual length (see pages 48–51).
- Detangle your curls with your fingers after applying conditioner to avoid breakage.

PERFECT PRODUCTS

- Co-wash shampoo (see page 24) and conditioners with a lot of slip
- Sliicone-free hair butters for moisture and definition

TIGHT COILS

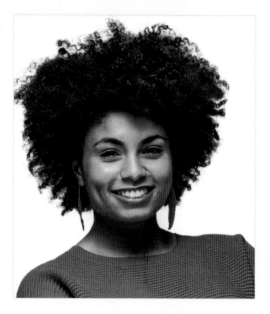

This is the most coarse of all curl types, and is highly susceptible to dryness and damage. The hair is tightly packed together, too, so it does not absorb or retain moisture easily. Tight coils also suffer from the highest amount of shrinkage (up to 75 percent of the hair's actual length).

QUICK TIPS

- Co-wash your hair to promote moisture, or opt for the "no-poo" method—dispense with shampoo and substitute apple cider vinegar, baking soda, or water to give your hair a break from chemicals.
- Use tea-tree-oil shampoo on the scalp only.
- Detangle your curls with your fingers after applying conditioner to avoid breakage.

PERFECT PRODUCTS

- Co-wash shampoo (see page 24) and deep conditioners with a lot of slip
- Deep-conditioning treatments

RESTORING YOUR NATURAL HAIR

"Transitioning" is the term used to describe hair that has previously been straightened, or relaxed, with chemicals and is now being allowed to return to its naturally curly state. New growth is left to emerge without chopping off any previously relaxed hair. This is a wise route to go if you want to return to your natural hair without sacrificing any length; you are free to let your natural hair grow at its own pace. However, during this process, you are dealing with two different hair textures—the relaxed part and the emerging natural new growth. Luckily, there are several things you can do to keep your hair looking its best.

PUT A HALT ON CHEMICAL TREATMENTS

During this time it's best to avoid any chemical treatments. Hair is made drier and more prone to breakage with a relaxer, so any additional chemical treatments will damage the hair even more. As transitioning to natural hair can be a long, grueling process, keep your styling options open by trying wigs and clip-in extensions to change it up instead.

HEALTHY HAIR-CARE ROUTINE

From shampoo to styling, you'll want to create a healthy routine that will give your hair the best possible outcome. Choose products and protein treatments that will encourage strength and elasticity. A moisturizing shampoo and conditioner are key basics. Deep conditioning is also crucial, and should be done with every wash.

CHOOSE PROTECTIVE STYLING

Low-manipulation, protective styling is another key tool. Any chemically treated hair is already weak and damaged, and manipulating it excessively can stall the growing process altogether. Give your hair a break by using protective styles during the week, such as buns, braids, or twists, and by keeping your hands out of your hair. You can also opt for twist-outs, which can last up to five days.

REGULAR TRIMS

As much as we dislike losing length, in the name of healthy hair it is so worth it. Say goodbye to those awful, damaged ends by having your hair trimmed regularly. For most hair types, the general recommendation is three months, but consult with your stylist to find what is best in your case.

PROTEIN TREATMENTS

Not all protein treatments are the same, so it's a good idea to consult a professional. If your hair is both color-treated and relaxed, you need to use a protein treatment that strengthens the hair, and then follow up with moisturizing products to bring back the elasticity. Note, though, that using too much protein can give hair a stiff and crunchy feel.

OILS

When styling hair, be sure to seal it with an oil for better moisture retention. Different oils offer different benefits, so think about which ones might best suit your needs. Coconut oil can be used to moisturize and seal the hair. It can penetrate the hair shaft easily, making it an ideal choice for regular use. Although they don't penetrate as deeply as coconut oil, olive and argan oil are also both great sealants that penetrate the hair shaft. If you want an oil solely for sealing purposes and to add shine, try jojoba oil. For more on oils, see pages 24–25.

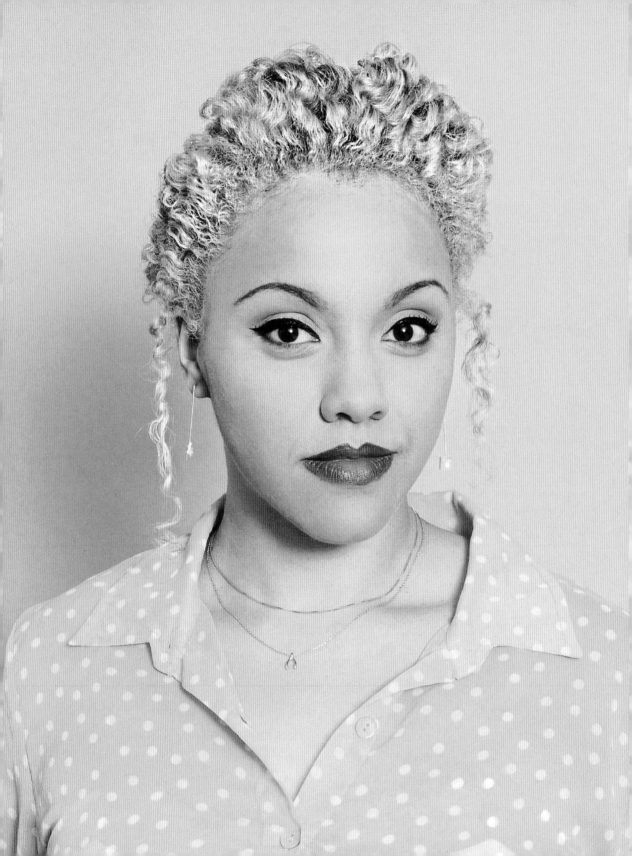

PERMED AND COLOR-TREATED HAIR

PERMED HAIR

Perms should always be done by a professional. As with any chemical treatments that alter the state of your hair, you need to do your research. Look for a salon that offers the service and make plans to speak with a stylist before making any hasty decisions. Discuss the pros and cons with them beforehand, so that you know exactly what you're getting your hair into.

Before you have your hair permed, have your ends trimmed. Hair should be in a healthy state before any chemical treatments are carried out. Split ends can travel up the hair shaft, causing further damage.

CARING FOR YOUR PERM

Avoid washing your hair immediately after a perm, while the chemicals may still be doing their work; wait at least two days before you shampoo to avoid losing the curl pattern.

Scrunch your hair while wet and use moisturizing curl-defining products for the best results. You should also deep-condition with every wash for soft, healthy, manageable curls.

SCRUNCH AWAY

When styling permed hair, be sure to scrunch your wet strands and use a foaming mousse to hold the curl. Use a product that contains humectants, which naturally draw moisture from the environment into the hair. If you have drier, denser curls, use moisturizing styling milk for shine and better wearability. You can also seal your curls with jojoba oil to retain moisture (see page 24).

COLORED HAIR

As with a perm—or any chemical process—you want to make sure you are replenishing the moisture that sometimes gets lost when you color your hair, so always stick to moisturizing products. A professional should be able to advise you.

USE COLOR-SAFE PRODUCTS

Permed and color-treated hair are very similar to hair that has undergone the relaxing process, so you must use shampoos and conditioners that restore the hair's health and flexibility.

With colored hair, always use color-safe products. This will prolong the life of your color and make it possible for you to go for longer periods of time in between touch-ups.

LEFT: Messy French twist, page 170

ESSENTIAL PRODUCTS

PRODUCTS FOR CLEANSING AND CONDITIONING

While every girl's needs differ when it comes to hair care, there are some essentials that we all need to have in our bathroom cabinet!

SHAMPOO

Contrary to what you may have heard, shampoo can be a healthy part of a curly girl's hair routine. Choose one that caters to your specific hair type. Universally, you want to look for products that are free from drying agents such as sulfates, which contain chemicals that can derail your healthy hair journey. Your shampoo should clean the scalp and dissolve any buildup without stripping the hair of vital oils and nutrients. Your hair should feel clean afterward, but not brittle and dry. Start with a quarter-sized portion, and scale up the amount if you have very long or thick hair. If you can achieve a good lather you are using plenty! Unless you are using a shampoo designed for daily use, leaving at least a day or two between washes will prevent any unwanted dryness.

CO-WASH

A co-washing shampoo cleanses the hair in the most moisturizing way possible. While this can be done using a regular conditioner, there are also co-washing shampoos that have been formulated to mimic the qualities of a shampoo by removing dirt and debris, but without the drying after-effects. Co-washing increases elasticity and provides a lot of slip, which makes the washing process easier for drier, coarser hair. It is also great for scalp health. Co-wash as often as you feel you need to, and check the product details for the correct amount to use.

CLARIFYING SHAMPOO

Clarifying shampoos work hard to deep-clean the scalp and remove a buildup of dirt and oil gathered from both hair products and the environment. Even the best shampoos can leave a film on your hair, so a clarifying shampoo will achieve that extra-clean feeling. Use the same amount as for a regular shampoo, but restrict usage to once a month.

CONDITIONER

This is one of the most important parts of your routine. The goal is to slide through the ridges of the hair and cater to those small spaces that are dense and go without attention. Unlike straight hair, the ridges in curls can prevent natural oils from traveling down the hair shaft and moisturizing the rest of the hair. Use a conditioner matched to your hair type, and use a deep-conditioning treatment regularly for soft, shiny, manageable hair. In both cases, use enough product to coat all of your hair.

HAIR MASKS / RECONSTRUCTORS

Hair masks are essential for all curl types. Some focus on deep conditioning and revitalizing curls, others work to strengthen the hair with protein, and some even reconstruct damaged hair, so choose one that meets your needs. Once a week is frequent enough for this sort of treatment, but be guided by the condition of your hair.

OILS

You can use hair oils as a moisturizer, as a moisture sealant, or to aid detangling your hair prior to shampooing. The best ones to have on hand are coconut, olive, argan, and jojoba. Coconut and olive oil are rich moisturizers and can make a much easier job of detangling coarse hair. Argan and jojoba oil are lighter in texture, add a natural luster to the hair, and work well as sealants. Jojoba oil mimics sebum, an oil that is naturally produced by the scalp, which makes it perfect as a scalp moisturizer, too. With oil, you need only a small amount—warm up a few drops in your hands and work it through your curls as needed.

JAMAICAN BLACK CASTOR OIL

This is derived from castor beans and is rich in omega-9 fatty acids, which help moisturize the scalp. Just a few drops rubbed into the scalp at night or after cleansing can promote growth and help repair split ends.

LEAVE-IN CONDITIONER

For curlier, thicker hair types, a leave-in conditioner lotion or cream is ideal. This type of conditioner also works wonders on chemically treated hair—think relaxed, colored, and permed hair. The leave-in will replenish moisture and help curls revert to their natural state. If you've been flat-ironing your hair frequently and are suffering from heat damage, a good leave-in will also help revive your curl pattern. Don't apply more than you need, though, or it may weigh down your hair.

LEAVE-IN SPRAY CONDITIONER

Dull curls need to be revived every few days, and a good leave-in spray will do just that. Keep a moisturizing leave-in spray for second- or third-day hair. You can also use it after you shower, right before you style.

PRODUCTS FOR STYLING

For most styling purposes, try to have the following on hand before you begin.

CURL DEFINER

A curl definer or styling lotion helps to control frizz, add moisture, and provide curls with a manageable hold. It can be used on wet or dry hair, so it is a very versatile styling tool. For simplicity I recommend this product for a lot of the tutorials later in this book, but make sure you choose a definer that suits your hair type and meets your styling needs. Alternatively substitute it for something that has been proven to work better for your hair type.

For finer, wavier hair types, mousse might be a better option because it won't weigh down the hair as much. For curlier textures, a styling milk or lotion will provide medium hold without having a crunchy after-effect. If you prefer a little more hold, add a lightweight gel to the hair after applying curl definer, then seal with an oil to enhance the shine. Coarser, denser hair types can also try butters and gelées for moisture and hold.

FOAMING MOUSSE

Foaming mousse works on a multitude of curl types. Use a water-based mousse alone or with your styling milk for better product absorption and hold. Foaming mousse is great for wet, curly hair, but it can also be helpful when curling your hair using a heat-free method (see pages 44–51).

HAIRSPRAY

One of the oldest styling products around, and still one of the best! A few squirts of hairspray will keep most styles intact all day long. Modern formulas offer plenty of hold without any stickiness. However, the fumes can be strong, so don't use more than you need, and make sure you apply it in a well-ventilated room.

HAIR SERUM

Hair serum is a thick, silicone-based product that coats the hair to give it extra shine. It is the best product to use for dealing with flyaways. You need to use only a small amount.

ESSENTIAL TOOLS

TOOLS YOU USE

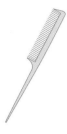

RAT-TAIL COMB

This tool has a fine-toothed comb at one end and a thin handle at the other end. The comb can be especially useful for backcombing, while the handle end can be used to section hair by creating a neatly defined part.

MICROFIBER TOWEL

A microfiber towel is one of the best tools to have on hand when drying your curls. It absorbs water quickly and is much gentler on your hair than an ordinary towel. Regular towels can damage the hair's cuticle, which leads to frizzy hair, but microfiber towels are made from a much smoother material. Because of its amazing ability to soak up water, it will also cut down blow-drying time. (If you want healthy hair, you should consider using as little heat as possible in your daily routine.)

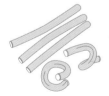

FLEXI RODS

These are the perfect tool for creating curls without heat (see pages 44–45). They are much easier to use than old-fashioned plastic curlers, and they are available in several sizes. Flexi rods are flexible, light, and comfortable enough to leave in overnight.

SCALP MASSAGER

Scalp massagers promote growth by lubricating the scalp, while helping to prevent flaking. Our hair naturally secretes oils, and massaging the scalp helps to move oil down the hair shaft which helps to moisturize and protect the hair. It also helps soothe the scalp and make the hair more resilient.

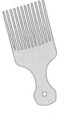

BLOW-DRYER WITH DIFFUSER

Blow-drying your curls with a diffuser attachment will cut down drying time, reduce frizz, and give you lustrous curls. Diffusers help blow-dryers distribute the air less aggressively, which stops frizz. The key is to diffuse large sections of hair at a time, diffusing at the ends, facing the attachment up toward your head. Use your fingers to gently scrunch hair and assist curl definition. Use the cool setting to avoid heat damage.

HAIR PICK

The widely spaced, long teeth of a hair pick are perfect for working down through very curly hair and lifting curls at the roots.

RIGHT: Mini side twists, page 174

WIDE-TOOTHED COMB

This should be in every curly girl's kit. The wide spaces make it an ideal tool for gentle detangling, and the width of the bristles won't cause friction and damage your hair. Combs with tightly packed bristles should be avoided if possible. Use your wide-toothed comb to fluff the roots of second-day or freshly blow-dried hair, to part hair, and to detangle.

SILK OR SATIN PILLOWCASE

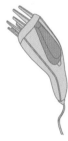

While you rest, so should your hair. When we sleep we have a tendency to toss and turn, and sleeping for eight hours on cotton can cause friction, frizz, and dryness. Try using a silk or satin pillowcase instead to protect your curls while you're asleep. Alternatively, tuck your curls away in a silk or satin bonnet.

HAIR STEAMER

Hair steamers use moist heat on the hair, which aids in restoring and retaining moisture. Steamers can strengthen the hair and improve elasticity, too. You can use a hair steamer to help loosen any tangles, and also during deep-conditioning—the steamer will open up the cuticles, enabling better product absorption. Use a steamer throughout the week to refresh and moisturize, and you will see a difference in your curls.

TOOLS YOU WEAR

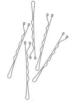

BOBBY PINS

Always keep lots of pins on hand—you'll need them for most of the styles in this book. Even though they can't match hair ties for strength, they are kinder to the hair, so substitute them whenever possible.

HAIR TIES

A true essential—there is no limit to the number of styles you can create with the help of the humble hair tie! Choose ties that will slip over your hair easily without snagging. You may also want to seek out some clear elastic ties. These will not last as long as regular hair ties, but they are great for styles that call for a bit of subtlety!

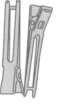

HAIR CLIPS

Hair clips make styling your hair easy-peasy. They come in a range of sizes, but are always long and wide enough to hold whole sections of hair out of the way while you work on other sections.

RIGHT: Cinnamon roll
braid, page 162

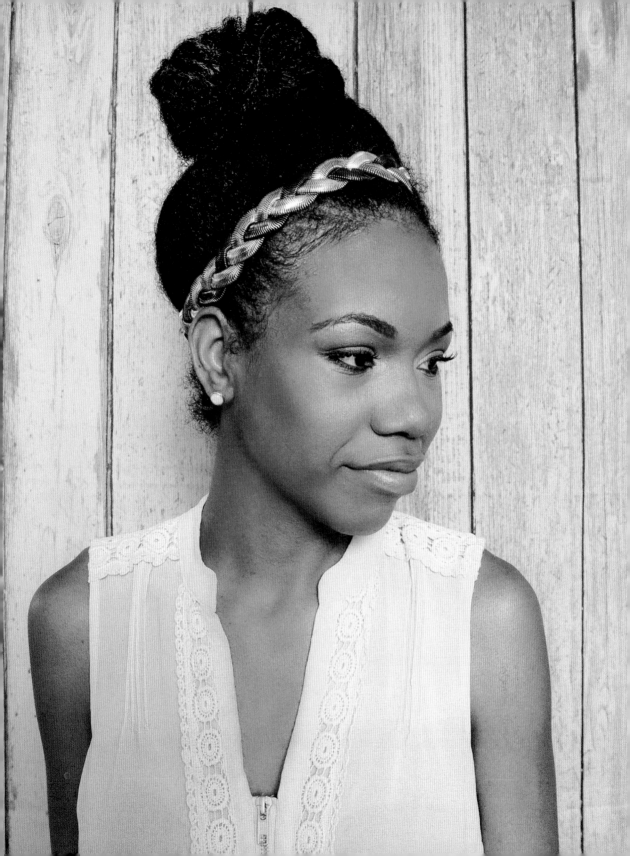

WASHING ROUTINE

A proper washing routine is a must. You will obviously need to choose products that suit your particular hair type, but I recommend detangling your hair with either oil or conditioner prior to shampooing. Detangling will make the washing process much easier. It can be done on wet or dry hair, and the choice of product will depend on your hair's condition.

DETANGLING WITH OIL

If your hair tends to be very dry and prone to severe tangling, try detangling with coconut or olive oil on dry hair. Oil will provide plenty of slip and make the task a lot quicker.

Start by sectioning your hair into four equal parts and secure each section with a hair clip. Working from the back to the front, take down your first section and massage your chosen oil through it. Work your way up from the ends of the hair toward the scalp, gently separating the strands as you go. As mentioned earlier, a steamer can soften the hair and allow the oil to penetrate more deeply. Once your first section feels sufficiently detangled, re-clip it and move on to the next section. Continue to massage oil into each section in turn. Rinse with cool water once you have finished.

DETANGLING WITH CONDITIONER

If your hair is in good shape and requires only a light detangling, you can use conditioner on wet hair. Soak your hair thoroughly with cool water and add a generous amount of conditioner all over. For looser curl types, glide your fingers through your curls from the roots to the ends. For thicker, coarser hair, it can be easier to divide the hair into sections once it has enough slip, and then work through each section, slowly separating and working in the product. Rinse with cool water once you have finished.

WASHING

First select a cleaning product that will not only remove dirt, oil, and buildup, but will promote moisture and revive your curls too. If your hair needs cleansing, you can use shampoo. If dryness is an issue, you can substitute a co-wash (page 24) or conditioner. Where you wash your hair is completely up to you. It can be done in or out of the shower.

Make sure your hair is competely soaked through after detangling. This will distribute other products more effectively and allow for better penetration. Massage the cleanser all over your scalp with your fingers. Massaging the scalp should be done for at least five minutes of every wash. This will cure flakiness, stimulate growth, and cleanse the scalp.

Now thoroughly rinse away all of the cleaning product and follow up with your conditioner of choice. If you struggle with moisture retention, you can steam your hair once again to allow better penetration of the conditioner. Rinse thoroughly to finish.

RIGHT: Boho fishtail, page 158

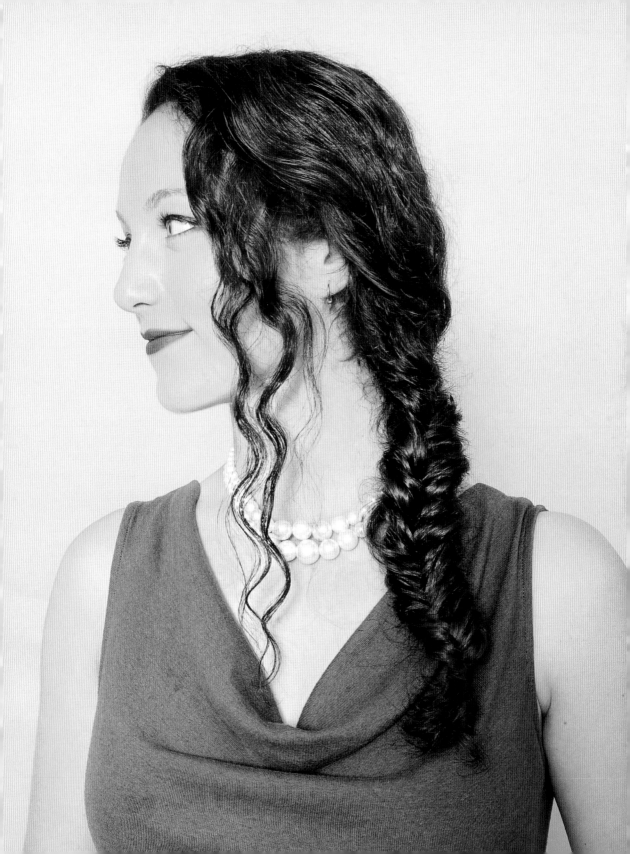

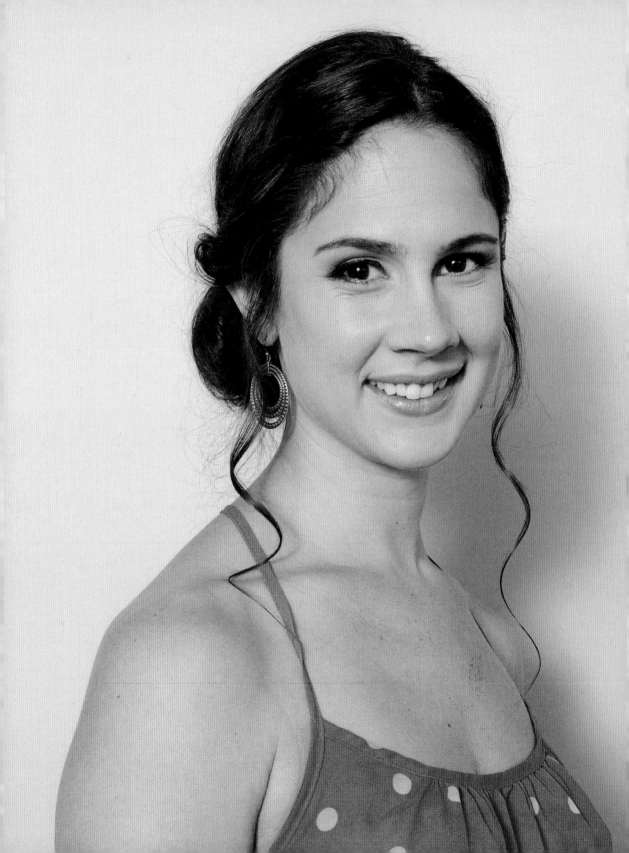

DRYING ROUTINE

USING A MICROFIBER TOWEL

Heat can be damaging to the hair, so it's good to air-dry your curls as often as possible. You can speed up this process, though, by absorbing any excess water from your hair with a microfiber towel. This will allow you to soak up moisture without rubbing against the hair shaft and irritating the cuticle. Squeeze at the roots first, to move the water downward, then slowly squeeze your way toward the ends of your hair. Your hair should be damp but not wet.

Now apply a leave-in product and styler of your choice. Using your fingers, rake the product throughout your hair. Work from the roots to the ends and, once you are done, gently scrunch your hair to encourage a more prominent curl.

If you have time to let your hair dry naturally, this is all you need to do. You may also opt to proceed with styling while your hair is still wet—plenty of the tutorials later in this book are suitable for both wet and dry hair.

T-SHIRT METHOD

A cheap and effective alternative to a microfiber towel is an old T-shirt. Slide your hair into the opening of a clean T-shirt and then twist it to squeeze out excess water. If you choose to air-dry your curls, you can wear the T-shirt on your head while doing your makeup and other morning chores. Then, when you're ready to style, simply remove the T-shirt, add some curl definer, style, and you're ready to go!

BLOW-DRYING

Although you need to avoid heat wherever possible, there will be times when this isn't practical. However, as long as it's done with care, the damaging effects of blow-drying can be kept to a minimum.

Start by absorbing excess water with a microfiber towel, as described above. Then select your hair dryer's cool setting, in combination with a diffuser attachment. Gently scrunch your curls as you hold the attachment over them, taking care not to linger in one place for too long. Your hair doesn't need to be bone dry, either. You can blow-dry until your hair is almost dry and then let nature complete the job!

LEFT: Twisted chignon, page 100

NATURAL REMEDIES

APPLE CIDER VINEGAR

Apple cider vinegar is no longer just for salad dressing! It serves as a great natural hair rinse. Every now and then your hair will suffer from a layer of buildup that even a great shampoo can't get rid of. Try rinsing with half a cup of apple cider vinegar to remove even the toughest product buildup.

AVOCADO

If you want to go more green, avocados are a great place to start. Instead of using a leave-in conditioner, opt for an avocado hair mask. This "superfood" is filled with protein, vitamins, and amino acids that help bring curls back to life. If you're suffering from damage due to chemical treatments or heat, add a little raw egg to the mix and you've got the perfect reconstructing treatment. Try using this once a week. The mixture won't keep, though, so make a fresh batch each time—half an avocado and a couple of teaspoons of egg is plenty for medium-length hair.

FLAXSEED GEL

Flaxseed gel helps with the moisture, growth, and health of curly hair, and provides hold without any "crunch." It is made from flaxseeds and aloe vera. For an affordable way of creating definition without the use of harsh chemicals, try making your own. Boil two cups of water and half a cup of flaxseed in a pot. Stir the mixture with a wooden spoon until it begins to thicken and froth (about ten minutes). Turn the heat down and stir until a jelly has formed, then remove the pot from the heat and pour the jelly through a strainer. As it cools, whisk in a tablespoon of aloe vera gel. When it is nice and smooth, transfer it to an airtight container and store it in the fridge. It should last for a couple of weeks.

HUMIDIFIERS

The harsh winter months can wreak havoc on our hair. A humidifier moistens dry air, making it an ideal natural remedy for curly hair. Unlike nature's humidity, which tends to cause frizz, this device balances out the moisture in a room. Plug in a humidifier in your bedroom so that it works while you sleep—you'll notice its benefits immediately.

OLIVE AND COCONUT OIL

These rich oils are excellent for detangling thick, coarse hair. They also smooth the outer cuticle of the hair and penetrate the shaft to help retain moisture. Warm a tiny amount of oil in your hands and work it through dry hair before styling. Or use it as a conditioner—leave it in for 20 minutes, or even overnight, before washing with shampoo. A weekly hot-oil treatment can be great for conditioning, too (see page 38).

OMEGA-3

Need a shine boost? Incorporate some omega-3 fatty acids into your diet. Some of the best sources of this are oily fish (such as salmon and mackerel), flaxseeds, and chia seeds. Omega-3 is great for treating dry scalp conditions. It also strengthens the hair, and can help those suffering from hair loss.

YOGURT

Yogurt is packed with proteins and nutrients. The lactic acid and zinc act as natural hydrators for dry, damaged hair, aiding scalp health and strengthening hair follicles. Whip up a weekly deep-conditioning treatment using 2 tablespoons of plain yogurt and an egg to add luster to dull curls.

RIGHT: Crown braids, page 156

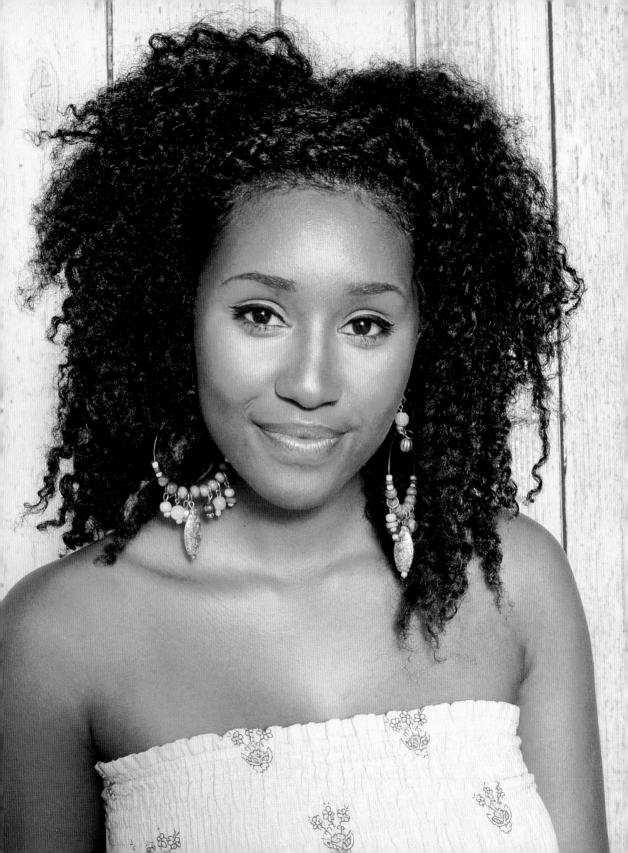

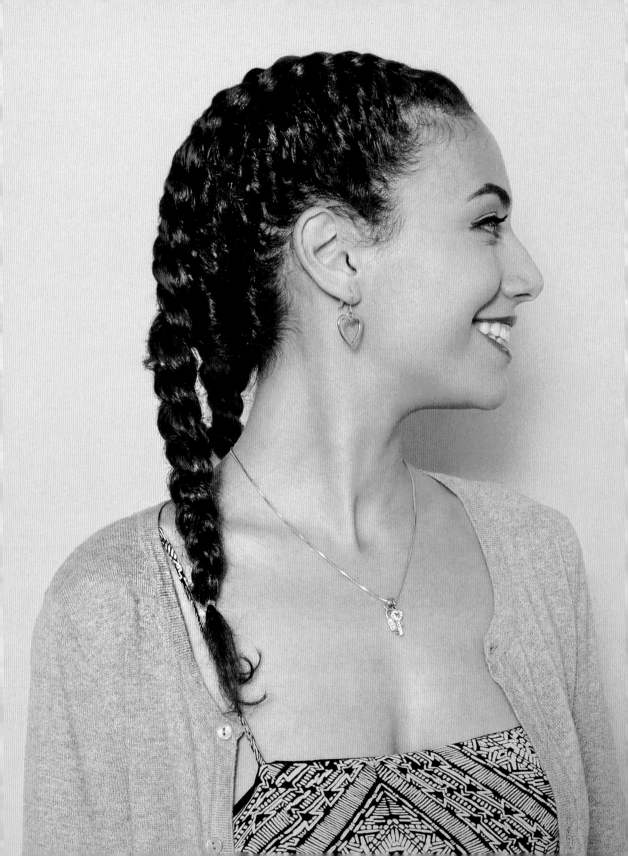

FINDING A GOOD HAIRDRESSER

We have all been there: needing a trim with no one to call. Finding a good hairdresser can seem like a daunting task, but it is necessary in order to keep your hair always looking its best. Hairdressers and stylists study hair professionally and can recommend products that cater to your specific needs. They can also spot split ends from a mile away. Here are some quick pointers for finding that perfect salon.

CHECK OUT YOUR NEIGHBORHOOD

There's nothing more comforting than needing a trim or color checkup and having a reliable stylist nearby. If there is a salon close to where you live, pay it a visit—go inside, browse the aisles, and spend a bit of time speaking with a few stylists to feel it out. The atmosphere should be warm and comfortable and make you feel at ease.

LOOK ONLINE

The Internet is chock-full of salons to choose from. Go online and check out the salons that are close to home. It's great to have options when choosing a hairdresser, as they all offer different services. Consider those that might be close to work, too.

Going online to find a hairdresser can also score you deals when it comes to a haircut, color, or styling. There are all sorts of deals available online, and who knows—that one deal might land you in the chair of a hairstylist you really love.

HOW KNOWLEDGEABLE ARE THEY?

Your hairdresser should be professional and not only look the part, but have information to back it up. They should be aware of any precautions related to perms, relaxers, and colors, and should alert you to these before booking you for an appointment. They should also be able to analyze your hair type confidently and recommend products that will work for you.

LEFT: Dutch pigtails, page 168

AT-HOME HAIRDRESSING

KEEPING A ROUTINE

Practice makes perfect, as they say! Establishing a regular routine for your hair will ensure that you are maintaining a healthy regimen. You should always be aware of what your hair needs, and when. If you're a swimmer, for example, it can be beneficial to use a clarifying shampoo to lift the chlorine out of your hair and to compensate for any moisture loss with a deep conditioner once a week. If you struggle with damage generally, it can be helpful to add protein treatments to your weekly routine. Having a consistent routine will guarantee your hair is healthy, has strong growth, and is easy to manage.

DEEP-CONDITIONING MASKS

Treat yourself every now and again. At least once a week, it's great to pamper yourself and your hair with a good deep-conditioning mask. A little moisture boost will repair stressed hair and give it the TLC that it needs. If you straighten your hair frequently, you'll find that you have a harder time getting your curl to revert back to its natural pattern. A deep-conditioning treatment will soften your hair and help to reverse this problem.

You can make a conditioning mask at home (search online for recipes, or try one of the suggestions on page 34), or you can buy one from your local beauty-supply store or salon. Masks will usually need to be left on the hair for at least 10 minutes to penetrate thoroughly, but check your product for specific instructions. Thirty minutes is usually plenty.

HOT-OIL TREATMENTS

When it comes to dry hair you can't beat the benefits of oil. In addition to detangling and adding shine, they can be used for a luxurious weekly hot-oil treatment. Pour a few tablespoons of your favorite oil into a heat-safe container and warm it over a pot of boiling water for around 30 seconds. Take care, though—always check the temperature of the oil before applying it to your head. You need the oil to be hot but not scalding. Work the oil through your curls, then wrap your hair in a towel and relax for at least 10 minutes. Rinse thoroughly afterward.

HANDS-OFF STYLES

I can't stress enough how important it is not to overmanipulate your hair. Take your hands out of your hair and let it be! Constantly touching your hair, or styling it every day, can put unnecessary stress on hair that can eventually lead to a stunt in growth. Give your hair a break by wearing a protective style that lasts for a few days. There are plenty of options to choose from in this book.

COLORING

If you are planning to color your hair at home, proceed with caution. Most store-bought dyes contain drying agents that are extremely damaging to your hair. Good products are available, but make sure you do your research beforehand to address any possible issues.

RIGHT: Double Dutch braids, page 166

DOS AND DON'TS

DO:

Get timely trims

Treat yourself to a trim to get rid of straggly ends. If your ends are looking frayed and thin, it's time to give them a good snip! Split ends can cause knots and make the detangling process much harder than it should be. They will also travel up the hair shaft and stunt your hair's growth.

Different hair types grow at different rates, so pay attention to your growth pattern. Give yourself a length check regularly using a tape measure; this will help you notice if your ends are looking lifeless and uneven. Although trimming your hair will lead to a slight loss in length in the short term, it will prevent damage and benefit your hair in the long run.

Make the most of second-day hair

Second-day hair (even third-day) is a must for curly hair. Try to style your curls in the morning and then keep your hands out of your hair for the rest of the day, unless absolutely necessary. The less you manipulate your hair, the less stress you're putting on it. Revive your second- (or third-) day hair with a spritz of leave-in spray if it's a simple washed, curly style. If it's a twist-out, you will need to retwist your hair overnight or place your curls out of the way in a high ponytail. You can also tuck your curls into a silk or satin bonnet for extra overnight protection.

Refresh curls every few days

Water is your curls' biggest BFF! When your curls start to look dull, it's a sign that they need moisture. Spritz them with a mix of leave-in conditioner spray and water to soothe dehydrated strands. You can divide your hair into four sections and use fingers to distribute the mixture throughout your hair if it needs extra attention. If you are avoiding heat, allow your hair to air-dry.

Try the LOC or LCO method

The LOC method is a three-step way to add and retain moisture. LOC stands for "liquid–oil–cream," and indicates the order in which these products are applied. The liquid is generally a leave-in conditioner, used to hydrate the hair. This is followed by an oil to seal in the moisture, and finally a curl cream to close the hair cuticle and prevent moisture loss. The LCO method is the same, except in this case the second and third steps are swapped so that oil is used as a sealant at the end.

Both methods are applied to wet hair, and the three products used in combination will hydrate your curls and leave your hair soft and manageable. Stick to this regimen every time you wash your hair.

Use protective styling every week

As mentioned earlier, protective styling involves giving your hair a break from overstyling by wearing it in a style that can be preserved unchanged for a few days in a row. A bun, for example, can be worn for several days, while a more complex, "tighter" style, such as cornrows, flat twists, or braids, can last for even longer—up to five days. Generally, the longer the better.

Although you will want your style to be secure enough to last, do be gentle on your curls, and don't use styles that pull on the sensitive hairs along the hairline. Sleeping with a silk or satin bonnet or pillowcase will help your style stay fresh even longer.

DON'T:

Detangle dry hair . . .

...unless you pre-detangle it with oil first. If you're detangling your hair, the best way to do it is while wet. If you are pre-detangling, you can use your favorite oil as an aid (olive and coconut are great for this!). Massage the oil through, starting at the tips, and separate each curl with your fingers. Gently unravel the strands upward, toward the scalp. By the time you're finished, your hair should be nicely saturated and have a great slip.

Brush unnecessarily

Try to avoid brushing curly hair, unless you are using a detangling brush or blow-drying your hair straight. Brushing it is guaranteed to bring the frizz. If you need to tidy any stray hairs, use a comb instead.

Use two chemical processes at once

Curly hair is naturally drier than straight hair, so overloading on chemicals can cause damage and, occasionally, hair loss. If you are looking to have your hair permed, for example, and you also want to color it, speak to a professional stylist first. They may recommend choosing one or the other, or staggering the processes to limit damage.

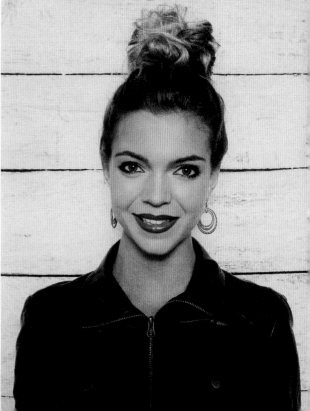

RIGHT: Top, Accent braids, page 176; Below, Messy bun, page 108

HEAT-FREE
CURLING
METHODS

FLEXI ROD METHOD

Using heat to curl your hair can cause damage over time, but luckily there are a number of heat-free curling techniques you can use instead. The next few pages offer three different methods for you to try: flexi rods, coiling, and twist-outs.

As the name suggests, flexi rods are flexible rollers used by curly and noncurly girls alike to create perfect bouncy curls. They are easy to work with—soft, lightweight, and bendy, capable of flexing into whatever shape you desire—which makes them a great choice for beginners. They also come in various sizes (measured by circumference), so you can select the size according to the curl you have in mind.

Wet hair is coiled around each rod, then released when dry to reveal bouncy, stretched curls. This technique can be used on all hair types, and it is a great way of stretching hair that normally curls up tightly. You can either leave your hair to air-dry or blow-dry it for quicker results.

1. Divide your hair into four equal sections and tie or clip each one up and out of the way. Now release one of the sections and give it some shine and moisture by applying a bit of your favorite curl definer and/or oil.

2. Grab a small strand of hair from this section and place it over the top of your first flexi rod to form your first curl.

3. Use one hand to hold the rod while you coil your hair around it with your free hand.

4. Keep wrapping your hair around the rod until you reach the ends. If you have trouble making the ends stick to the rod, add a little curl definer to the hair.

5. Once the hair is firmly wound around the rod, fold the rod in half and turn up the end with the hair on it, to prevent the hair from slipping off. Make sure the flexi rod is sitting securely against your head before moving on to the next strand. Complete this whole section of hair, then repeat Steps 1 to 5 for the other three sections.

When your hair is completely dry you can remove the rods. Once all of your curls have been released, you can create a bit of extra volume by carefully separating the curls and gently lifting the hair at the roots with a wide-toothed comb.

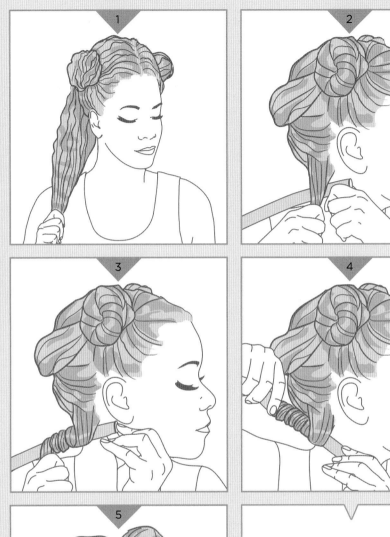

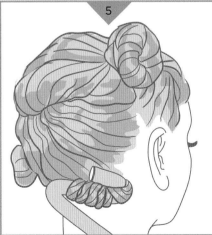

TOP TIP

Lifting the hair at the roots is not the same thing as backcombing, even though both techniques create volume. When you lift the roots, you are working in the same direction as your hair grows, not against it.

COILING METHOD

The coiling method is used to enhance ringlets and natural curls. A simple twisting motion is used on wet hair to create each curl. As your hair dries, it tightens to leave your curls in the shape of coils.

When coiling curly hair, always start with hair that is wet and has a nice slip to it. I generally use a leave-in conditioner, but you can also use a leave-in lotion, cream, or spray to achieve the right texture. After this, apply a curl definer and/or some gel to assist with hold. (Foaming mousse can also work well.)

You can wear coils for around five to seven days; just refresh your hair by spraying it with a mixture of water and leave-in conditioner every few days, and make sure you use a silk or satin hair bonnet or pillowcase at night to protect them. You can also wear your hair in a high ponytail during the day—a style that is often described as a "pineapple"!

1. Divide your hair into four sections and tie or clip each one up and out of the way. Take a small strand of hair from one of your bottom sections. This will be your first coil.

2. Begin twirling this strand of hair, using your pointer finger, making sure you twirl it thoroughly, from the roots to the ends.

3. When the strand has been completely twirled, use the fingers of one hand to hold it in its coiled state while you use the pointer finger of your other hand to coil the ends. You may find that you need to use a bit of water at this point—wetting the hair will make it more slippery and easier to coil.

4. Continue working in this way on strands taken from your first section of hair, making sure all the strands are the same size.

5. Complete the other three sections of hair in the same way until all your hair has been coiled. You can now leave your hair to air-dry, or you can blow-dry it using a diffuser attachment. When your hair is almost dry, massage some oil over your coils for shine and moisture retention.

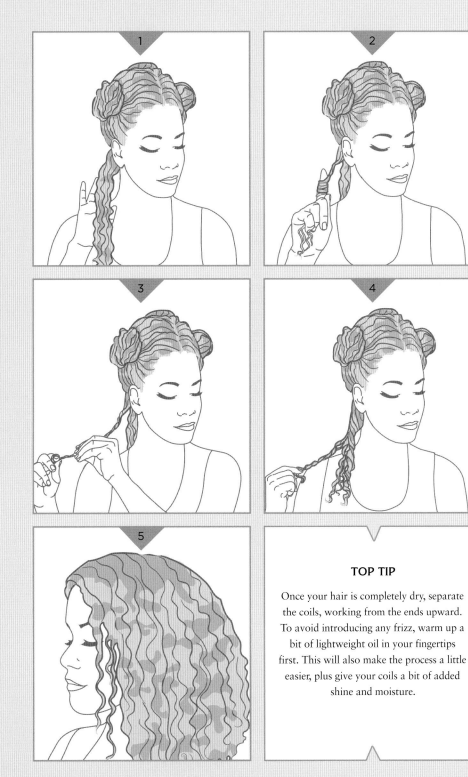

TOP TIP

Once your hair is completely dry, separate the coils, working from the ends upward. To avoid introducing any frizz, warm up a bit of lightweight oil in your fingertips first. This will also make the process a little easier, plus give your coils a bit of added shine and moisture.

TWIST-OUTS

Twist-outs are a great technique to use if you want to enjoy a new curl pattern. They are great for all hair types, creating a curl that can last for days. (You can also wear the twists themselves as a hairstyle. They will last for up to six days, which makes them a handy choice when you need to give your hair a break from styling.)

Results will vary depending on your hair type, but in all cases products are key. I generally use the LCO method as my go-to product technique (see page 40), but you can choose whatever products perform well for you when styling—styling paste, styling milk, lotion, custard, mousse, gel, and so on. You can create the twists on wet or dry hair, although if you have low-porosity hair, try twisting on dry hair. Leave the twists in for at least 8 hours for the best results (overnight is perfect), and if you start with wet hair, make sure your hair is completely dry before unraveling your twists.

Following are two different methods for achieving them: the two-strand method and the flat method (pages 50–51).

TWO-STRAND METHOD

This method creates a defined, wavy, stretched curl, so it is perfect if your hair curls tightly.

1. Begin by dividing your hair into four equal sections and secure each one using a hair tie or clip.

2. Release one of the sections and divide it in half. This will create medium-sized twists. Depending on the thickness of your hair and the size that you want for your twists, you might want to divide this section into three or four instead, but whatever you choose, make sure all your sections and subsections are the same size.

3. Pin one half of the section out of the way with a few bobby pins, then start work on the other half. Split it into two strands, then start twisting them together, left over right (or vice versa), until you reach the ends of the hair. You then have a few options. You can use mini hair bands to seal your ends, you can coil the ends with your fingers (if your hair is naturally curly); or you can use small hair rollers or flexi rods.

4. Remove the bobby pins from the second half of the section and create another two-strand twist in the same way.

5. Repeat this for the other three sections of hair until they are all twisted.

When it's time to release your twists, massage some lightweight oil onto your fingertips to help seal in moisture and prevent introducing any frizz as you work. Starting at the ends, slowly unravel each twist. The oil should make the untwisting process a bit easier. When all your twists have been unraveled, flip your head over and use a wide-toothed comb to lift your hair at the roots. You can also separate the strands if you want some extra volume. If you have fine hair, you may benefit from spritzing the roots with a bit of hairspray or root lifter.

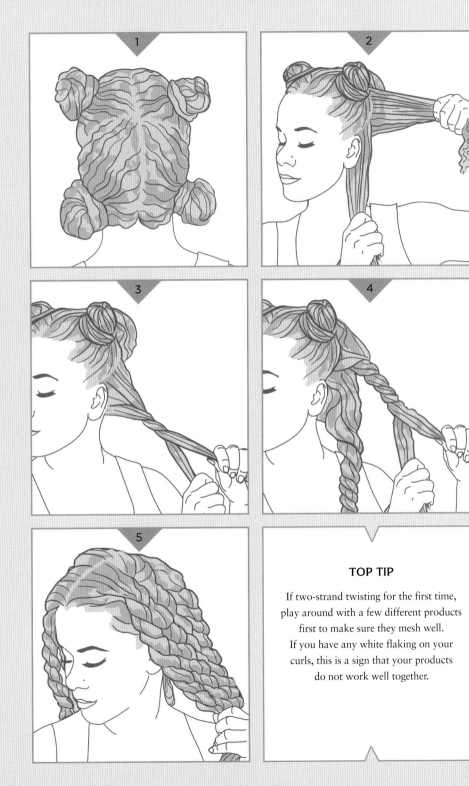

TOP TIP

If two-strand twisting for the first time,
play around with a few different products
first to make sure they mesh well.
If you have any white flaking on your
curls, this is a sign that your products
do not work well together.

FLAT METHOD

The flat twist-out routine is very similar to the two-strand method, but instead of hanging twists, this method produces twists that lay flat against the scalp, similar to a cornrow. As before, you can work with either wet or dry hair.

1. Divide your hair into four equal sections and secure each one with a hair tie or clip. Remove the hair tie from your first section and divide this in half. You may find it easier to begin with a section to the front, so that you can keep an eye on your work with this first set of twists, making sure they sit neatly against your scalp. As with the two-strand twist, make sure that your sections and subsections are all the same size, and as big or small as you want. The smaller the section, the smaller the twist.

2. Secure one half out of the way with some bobby pins while you begin on the other half. Starting at the beginning of your part, grab two strands from the section of hair you're working on and twist them, one over the other. After the first twist, grab some hair from along your hairline and add it into the strand on that side, feeding it into your twist. This is the same technique as used to create a French braid (see page 143), but here you are simply twisting rather than braiding.

3. Keep twisting and feeding in hair from either side as you go. Take your time, and use a mirror if necessary. Twist until you reach the ends of the hair, then coil the ends with your fingers (if your hair is curly), or secure them with a mini hair band or small roller.

4. Now release the second half of the section and create another twist in the same way. Again, take your time, making sure this second twist sits neatly in line with the first.

5. Repeat this process for the remaining three sections of hair until all of your hair has been twisted.

As with the two-strand method, when you are ready to release your twists, warm a little oil in your fingertips and then carefully unravel each twist. Finish by flipping your head over and using a wide-toothed comb or your fingers to lift your hair at the roots, applying a bit of hairspray or root lifter if needed.

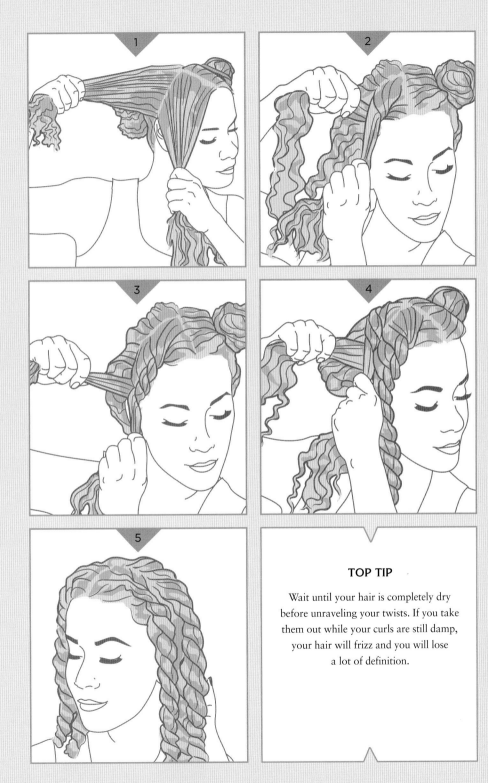

TOP TIP

Wait until your hair is completely dry before unraveling your twists. If you take them out while your curls are still damp, your hair will frizz and you will lose a lot of definition.

PONYTAILS

LOW PONYTAIL

BEST FOR
Medium to long hair

ACCESSORIES
Take this style up a notch
by accessorizing with a chic
headband or flower.

DIFFICULTY LEVEL
Easy

ASSISTANCE NEEDED?
No

The great thing about a low
ponytail is that you can keep it
simple and sporty, or dress it up
for a formal occasion. It's an easy
style for all hair types, but curly
hair is particularly good because
it adds so much extra shape and
dimension. This style is best for
medium to long hair, but it can
work well for shorter hair, too.

TRY THIS
This simple style can also be worn
off to the side (like the pony on
page 56), or with a middle part
(as shown on page 80). For
longer hair, you have the choice
of either swooping your curls over
your shoulders, or wearing them
hanging to the back.

SEE ALSO
Low curly side ponytail,
pages 56–57
Low ponytail with side
bangs, pages 82–83

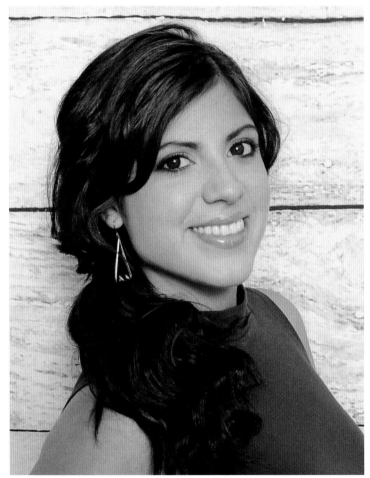

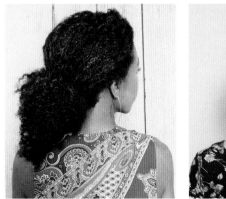

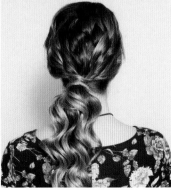

HOW TO DO IT

WHAT YOU NEED

- Curl definer
- Comb
- Hair tie
- Bobby pins
- Hairspray

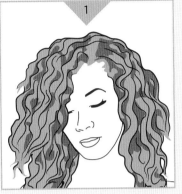

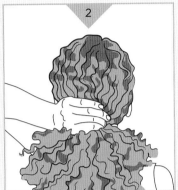

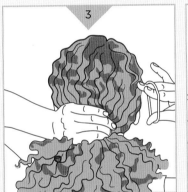

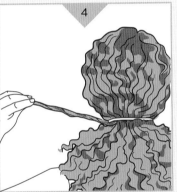

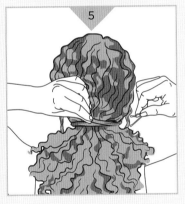

1. Second- or third-day dry hair is ideal for this style, since your curls naturally pick up more volume after a few days; otherwise apply some curl definer before you start.

2. Use a comb or your fingers to comb through your curls, then gather your hair at the nape of your neck.

3. Secure your ponytail with a hair tie.

4. Now separate out a small strand of hair from your ponytail.

5. Wrap this strand neatly around the hair tie and, when you have finished, tuck the end of it into the base of your ponytail and secure it with a couple of bobby pins. A light application of hairspray will then help keep everything in place.

TOP TIP

Whatever your curl type, you can enhance the curl in your ponytail by using the two-strand twist-out method (pages 48–49) the night before styling your hair.

LOW CURLY SIDE PONYTAIL

BEST FOR
Medium to long hair

ACCESSORIES
Jewelry for this style should be kept light and simple. A thin necklace or short, dangly earrings are all you need.

DIFFICULTY LEVEL
Easy

ASSISTANCE NEEDED?
No

Wearing your curls in a ponytail to the side is a simple and versatile choice, suited to all sorts of different occasions; it's also a surprisingly characterful, quirky look. This low ponytail suits any curl type, and it takes hardly any time at all.

TRY THIS
Since this style is flirty and simple, you'll find that natural makeup looks best. Try going for a liner on your eyes, paired with a bold lip color. Alternatively, combine a soft lip color with a slick of mascara.

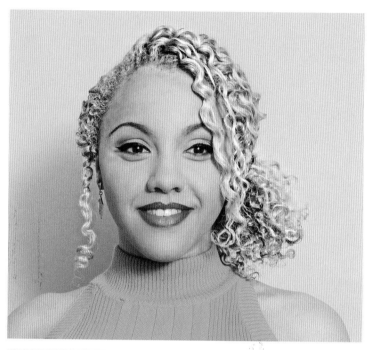

▶ **SEE ALSO**
Low ponytail, pages 54–55
Low ponytail with side bangs, pages 82–83

HOW TO DO IT

WHAT YOU NEED

- Comb
- Curl definer
- Hair tie
- Bobby pins
- Hairspray

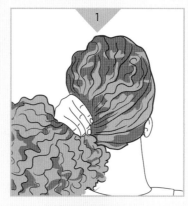

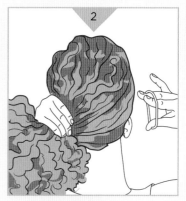

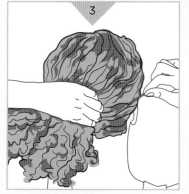

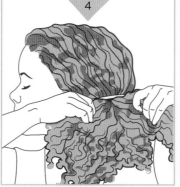

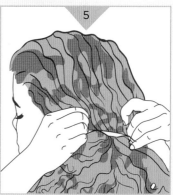

1. Smooth your hair toward the nape of your neck and to one side using a comb or your fingers. If you want to create a sleeker-looking ponytail, apply some curl definer before you start.

2. Secure your hair in place with a hair tie.

3. If you notice any stray hairs, simply tuck them in place and use bobby pins to keep them secure.

4. Grab your ponytail right at the base with both hands and wiggle it to create a bit more volume.

5. If you have thin hair, use your fingers to loosen the hair just above the hair tie, too. This will help create the illusion of thicker, more voluminous hair. Finish with a bit of hairspray for extra hold.

TOP TIP

Try two-strand-twisting your hair the night before creating this style (pages 48–49). Before you twist your hair, smooth some curl definer through it. When you remove the twists in the morning you will have the perfect hold and definition!

HIGH PONYTAIL

BEST FOR
Medium to long hair

ACCESSORIES
Bring more attention to your hair and facial features with a thick, shimmery headband. A solid headband is good for a more everyday look.

DIFFICULTY LEVEL
Easy

ASSISTANCE NEEDED?
No

This striking 'do is one of those styles that will really highlight your curl pattern. If your hair is tightly coiled and curls tightly after drying, you can always elongate your curls before you start by using the two-strand twist-out method (see pages 48–49). This will stretch your hair, giving you more length to work with, and a more dramatic pony!

TRY THIS
With a high ponytail, your hair is pulled away from your face, so make the most of this by accentuating your cheekbones with contouring powder, or your favorite blush and highlighter.

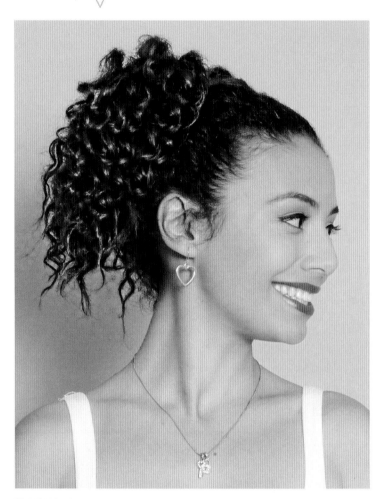

 SEE ALSO
High-crown ponytail, pages 62–63
Double ponytail, pages 66–67

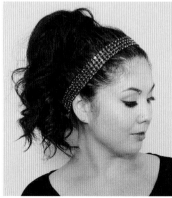

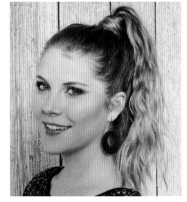

HOW TO DO IT

WHAT YOU NEED

- Curl definer
- Comb
- Hair tie
- Bobby pins
- Hairspray

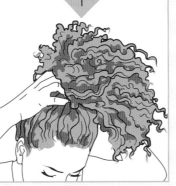

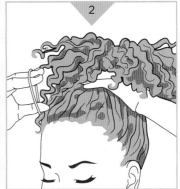

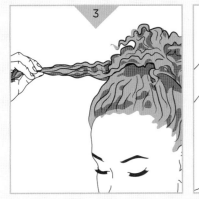

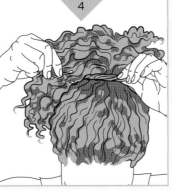

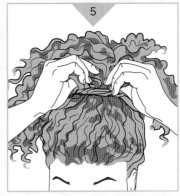

1. For high ponytails, second- or third-day hair is ideal. Your hair will be bigger and have more body, which will help with the success of this look. Start by flipping your hair forward, combing it toward the crown of your head, and hold it in place here. Adding curl definer will give it a smoother look.

2. Now loosen your grip slightly to create the appearance of thicker hair, and then secure your ponytail with a hair tie.

3. For extra detail and to create a sleeker finish, grab a small strand of hair from your ponytail and wrap it around the tie.

4. When you reach the end of the section, secure the end in place at the base of the ponytail using bobby pins.

5. Finally, lift the ponytail a bit at its base to create some height and extra volume. Apply hairspray to finish.

TOP TIP

If you have shorter hair, a neat trick is to tug gently at the hair at the rear of the ponytail—this will create the illusion of extra length. Or use the double ponytail method described on page 66 for an even longer-looking ponytail.

PONYTAIL FAUX HAWK WITH BRAIDS

BEST FOR
Medium to long hair

ACCESSORIES
This style provides plenty of interest by itself, but a glamorous statement necklace can take it to the next level. You can also enhance the hair itself by sliding a festive hair brooch into the base of the ponytail.

DIFFICULTY LEVEL
Hard

ASSISTANCE NEEDED?
Yes

A ponytail faux hawk combines a standard high ponytail and a faux hawk. The two Dutch braids on either side are a handy addition: They not only give you the hawk effect without having to commit to the full style, they also make the look much easier to re-create. This is the quintessential party hairstyle, so why not perfect it in time for your next big night out?

TRY THIS
Go for smoky eyes and a nude lip, or switch it up completely and create a clean look, with liner and mascara on the eyes, a defined brow, and a bright lip stain.

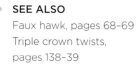

SEE ALSO
Faux hawk, pages 68–69
Triple crown twists,
pages 138–39

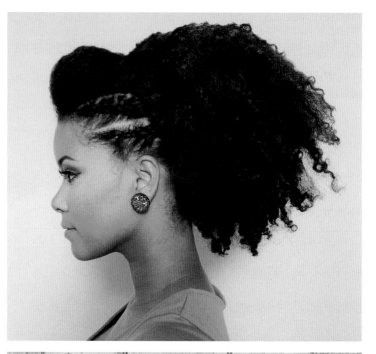

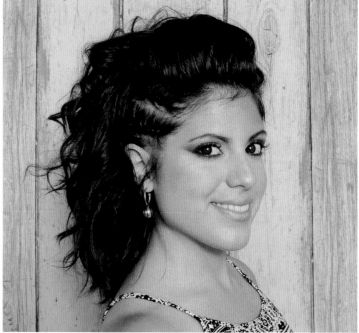

HOW TO DO IT

WHAT YOU NEED

- Comb
- Bobby pins
- Hair ties
- Hairspray (optional)

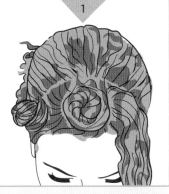

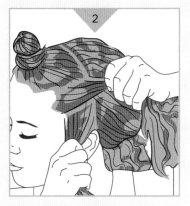

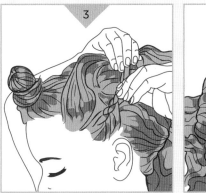

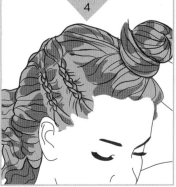

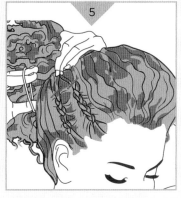

1. Using a comb separate out a rectangular section of hair, from one ear over to the other, then tie the rest of your hair out of the way. Divide the top section into three and coil two of these up.

2. Now divide the free-hanging section in half horizontally. Each of these two small sections will become a braid.

3. Working on the lower of the two sections, divide the hair into three strands and create a Dutch braid (see page 149 for instructions). Keep braiding until you get to the part, then use a pin to secure it. Repeat this with the second small section.

4. Now repeat Steps 2 and 3 on the opposite side of your head.

5. Release the central section and backcomb the roots. Lift and secure this hair with pins to create a pompadour. Finally, release the rest of your hair and lift it into a ponytail, incorporating the ends of your braids and pompadour. Secure with a hair tie.

TOP TIP

Spritz on a little hairspray while you are backcombing the pompadour. This will help it last much longer.

HIGH-CROWN PONYTAIL

BEST FOR
Medium to long hair

ACCESSORIES
Long feather earrings would make the best accessory for this dramatic-looking ponytail. Long jewelry softens and elongates the face.

DIFFICULTY LEVEL
Medium

ASSISTANCE NEEDED?
No

This ponytail creates the illusion of volume no matter how thick or thin your hair really is. To get the most out of this style, however, it is much better to start with dry, second- or third-day hair. Having curly hair is a definite bonus for this style, too, since curls naturally have a lot more body than straight hair.

TRY THIS
Since your hair is pulled away from your face, accentuate your features by adding definition to your eyebrows, filling them in with a brown pencil, and applying a contour color or blush to highlight your cheekbones.

SEE ALSO
High ponytail, pages 58–59
Double ponytail, pages 66–67

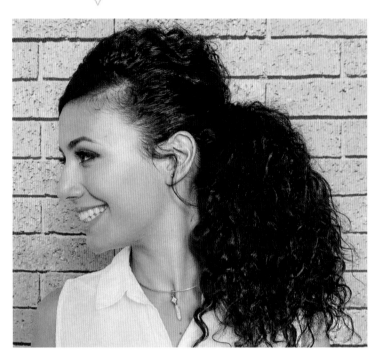

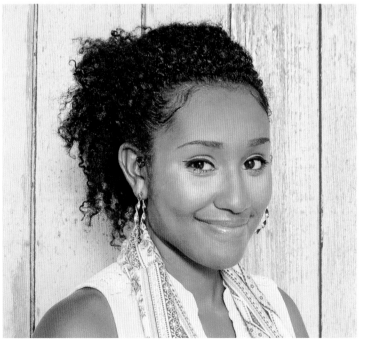

HOW TO DO IT

WHAT YOU NEED

- Comb
- Hairspray
- Bobby pins
- Hair tie
- Curl definer

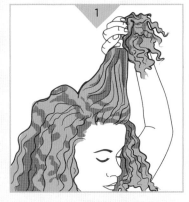

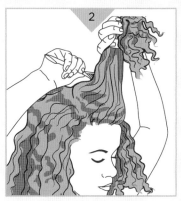

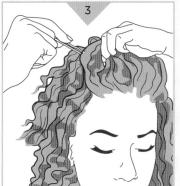

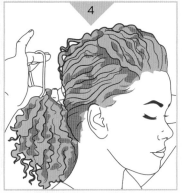

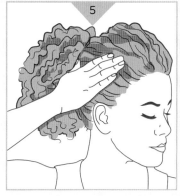

1. Use a comb to part out a large square section from the front of your head to the crown.

2. Backcomb this section from behind to create a bit more volume. If you have a looser curl type, use a little hairspray to hold the hair in place.

3. Once you have built up sufficient volume, lift up the middle of the section and use a few bobby pins to hold it in place here, securing it to the rest of your hair.

4. Now gather up the rest of your hair and create a low ponytail. Secure with a hair tie.

5. Smooth away any stray hairs with your fingers. Adding a little curl definer will hold them neatly in place.

TOP TIP

It's possible to hold any curl type in place with the help of a few bobby pins and some hairspray. However, a curl definer designed especially for curly hair is the best choice. It will keep stray hairs in place for a more polished look.

WRAPPED PONYTAIL

BEST FOR
Medium to long hair

ACCESSORIES
This is such a clean look that some chunky earrings are all you need to complete it.

DIFFICULTY LEVEL
Easy

ASSISTANCE NEEDED?
No

Wrapping a small section of hair around your ponytail gives it a much more polished look—you'll be amazed at how effectively you can jazz up your everyday ponytail just by adding this small detail. Longer, loose curl types can rock this style easily, and it also looks great in combination with the curly puff ponytail on page 74.

TRY THIS
The ponytail shown in the tutorial opposite is positioned at the back of the head, but you can play with the placement, placing it higher up, off to the side, or even in a half-up half-down style.

SEE ALSO
Low curly side ponytail, pages 56–57
High-crown ponytail, pages 62–63

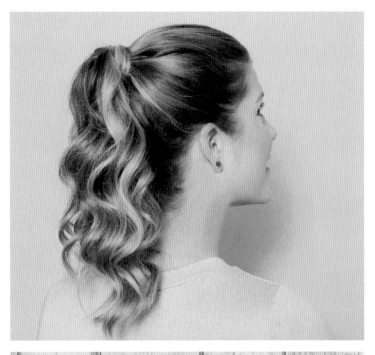

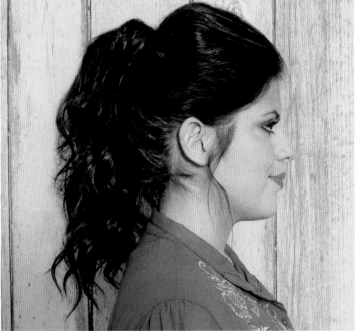

HOW TO DO IT

WHAT YOU NEED

- Hair tie
- Hair serum
- Bobby pins
- Hair pick or comb
- Curl definer (optional)

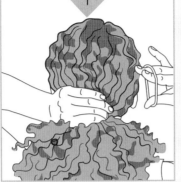

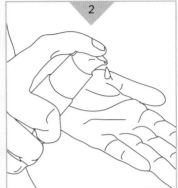

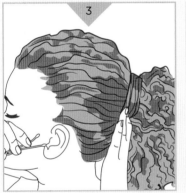

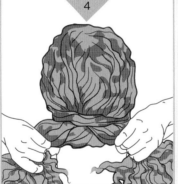

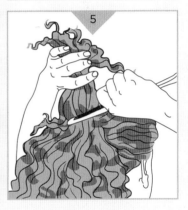

1. Gather your hair at your nape, and secure it with a hair tie.

2. It's a good idea to massage in a bit of hair serum along the hairline at this point for a sleeker finish, particularly if you have thick, frizzy hair. You can also use bobby pins to keep any stray hairs in place.

3. Now take a small strand of hair from your ponytail and wrap it around the hair tie. Slide bobby pins underneath the hair tie to secure it in place.

4. Tighten your ponytail by gently pulling the hair of your ponytail in opposite directions, taking care not to dislodge the base.

5. Finally, for some extra volume, take a pick or comb and lift the hair slightly at the base of the ponytail.

TOP TIP

You can make this look even more polished by adding a little bit of curl definer to your strand before wrapping it around your hair tie.

DOUBLE PONYTAIL

BEST FOR
All hair lengths

ACCESSORIES
Pair this pony with some pearl or shimmery stud earrings. Longer earrings will add even more glitz.

DIFFICULTY LEVEL
Easy

ASSISTANCE NEEDED?
No

This style can be flirty and fun, or simple and elegant. It works well with all hair lengths, but it is especially handy if you have short hair and want to create the illusion of extra length. The doubling up of the ponytails not only adds volume and dimension, it also creates the appearance of a longer ponytail than you could achieve with just a single ponytail.

TRY THIS
This hairstyle is simple and yet edgy, so a strong makeup statement can really complement it. Try a bold lip with natural eye makeup, or reverse this and go for smoky eyes combined with a nude lip.

SEE ALSO
High-crown ponytail, pages 62–63
Half-up half-down ponytail, pages 86–87

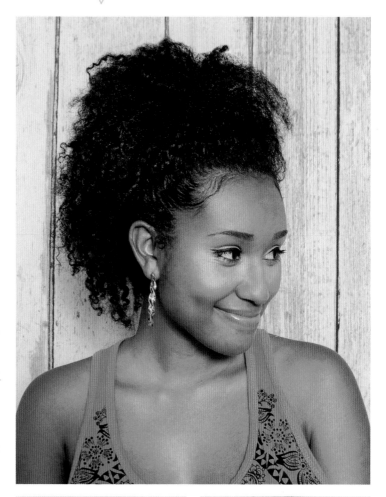

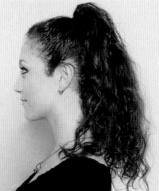

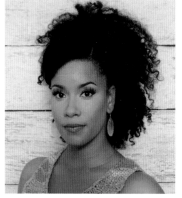

HOW TO DO IT

WHAT YOU NEED

- Curl definer
- Comb
- Hair ties
- Bobby pins
- Hairspray

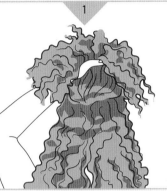

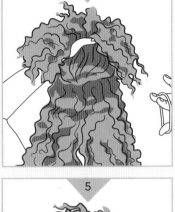

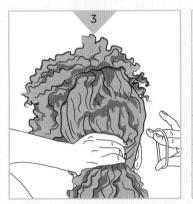

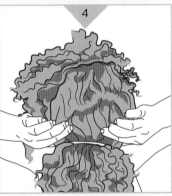

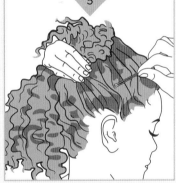

1. Apply a small amount of curl definer evenly through your curls, then section your hair in half, horizontally, using a comb.

2. Use a hair tie to secure the top half into a ponytail.

3. Use another hair tie to secure the bottom half.

4. Now loosen both the top and bottom ponytails a little with your hands, by wiggling the hair where it is held by the hair tie. This will have the effect of blending both ponytails together so they look like one long ponytail, instead of two.

5. Once you have the arrangement you want, hide the parting on either side of your head by adjusting the hair here and securing it with a bobby pin or two, then apply some hairspray to hold everything in place throughout the day.

TOP TIP

If you have bangs that are a little too short to reach the top ponytail, then simply sweep them off to the side instead and pin them in place, as demonstrated on page 103.

FAUX HAWK

BEST FOR
Short to medium-length hair

ACCESSORIES
Festive bobby pins along the sides of the faux hawk are a great addition to this killer style.

DIFFICULTY LEVEL
Medium

ASSISTANCE NEEDED?
No

The faux hawk is for bold, daring curly girls who want to have a little fun with their hair. You can wear this fab 'do just about anywhere, but I prefer to save it for festive occasions. Any hair length is fine, but since you'll be working with pins only, remember to have plenty on hand to keep everything secure. A faux hawk works best with thick, full curls, so you'll find it easiest to start with second- or third-day hair. Rocker chic has never looked so good!

TRY THIS
Pair this 'do with an effortless combo of smudged eyeliner and a bold lipstick that complements your skin tone.

SEE ALSO
Ponytail faux hawk with braids, pages 60–61
Halo bun, pages 96–97

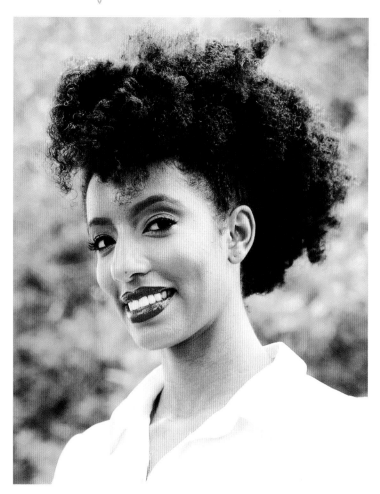

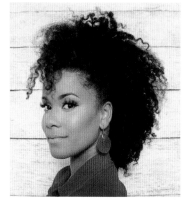

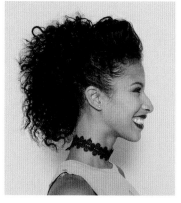

HOW TO DO IT

WHAT YOU NEED

- Curl definer
- Bobby pins

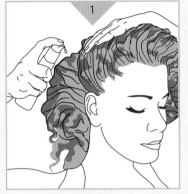

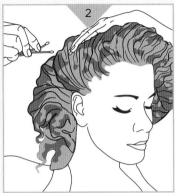

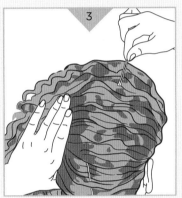

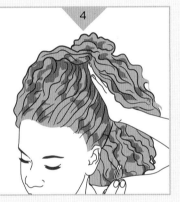

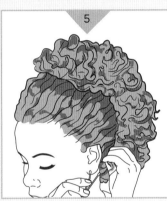

1. Massage some curl definer into your hair all the way around your hairline to smooth any stray hairs and flyaways.

2. Sweep your hair to one side and hold it in place here with one hand, then use your other hand to pin it down the center.

3. The pins can run all the way up the center of your head, in a vertical line up from the nape of your neck.

4. Once the first side is secure, flip your hair to the opposite side and repeat the same process, making sure you catch every last strand.

5. Check both sides are symmetrical and add any last pins for neatness and security. (If you have long hair and want to create the perfect faux hawk, simply fold the hair strands in half, then use bobby pins to keep them in place.)

TOP TIP

If your hair is particularly dense and heavy, crisscross your bobby pins for extra security. This technique will also save you a bit of time.

TWO-TWIST LOW PONYTAIL

BEST FOR
All hair lengths

ACCESSORIES
The intricate twists at the back are the highlight of this style. If you want to dress it up even more, add small stud earrings.

DIFFICULTY LEVEL
Hard

ASSISTANCE NEEDED?
No

This style is simple and yet oh so elegant. The tutorial opposite demonstrates how to create a pronounced bouffant, but this can be as dramatic or as subtle as you like, as seen in the variations on this page. Either way, this method of creating a raised crown using a small bun is a good option if you feel like your hair needs a break from backcombing. It can be much quicker, too!

TRY THIS
Why not try adding in swooped bangs? Part a small square section on top for this, pin it behind your ears, and then continue with the steps as described opposite.

SEE ALSO
Double-twist side ponytail, pages 76–77
Twisted half-up ponytail, pages 78–79

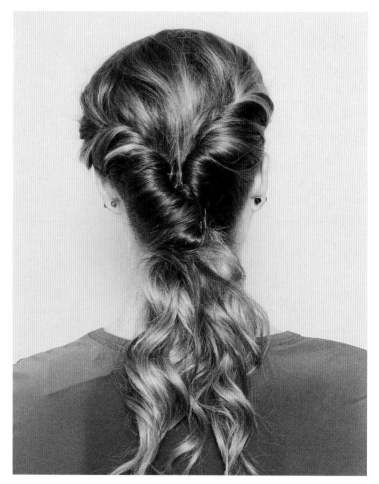

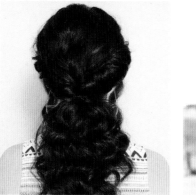

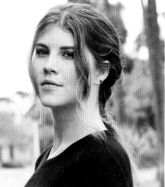

HOW TO DO IT

WHAT YOU NEED

- Comb
- Hair ties
- Bobby pins

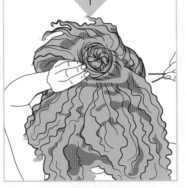

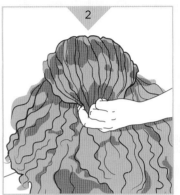

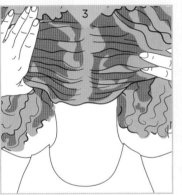

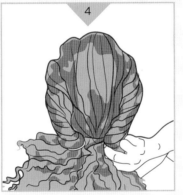

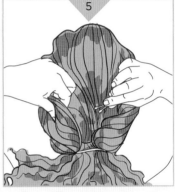

1. First off you need to create the bun to support the lifted crown. Separate out a small section at your crown with a comb, form a ponytail with it, then wrap the ponytail around the hair tie in a bun shape. Secure this with a few bobby pins.

2. Now gather your hair from the front and side of your face and smooth it over the top of the bun. Play with this until you have the desired raised-crown shape, then secure it with a few pins.

3. Now divide the rest of your hair vertically into two equal halves. Tie up one half and place it off to the side for now.

4. Working with the other half, begin twisting the hair down toward the nape of your neck. Once you reach the nape, secure it into a ponytail. Repeat this with the other half.

5. Finally, use a hair tie to combine both ponytails.

TOP TIP

To avoid a wide gap in between the twists, lift and pull each twist toward the center and secure it with extra bobby pins.

ROPE PONYTAIL

BEST FOR
Medium to long hair

ACCESSORIES
Long earrings and a flower headband are perfect partners for this pony.

DIFFICULTY LEVEL
Easy

ASSISTANCE NEEDED?
No

The rope style will liven up your standard ponytail in a few easy steps. It adds dimension, can be worn on any occasion, and is perfect for those times when your hair is not cooperating and you simply want to keep it away from your face. You can also wear this style wet or dry.

TRY THIS
Match this style's simplicity with a fun and pretty look—a subtly contoured eye with a touch of mascara, and a soft color for both lips and cheeks.

▶ **SEE ALSO**
Double ponytail, pages 66–67
Bubble ponytail, pages 92–93

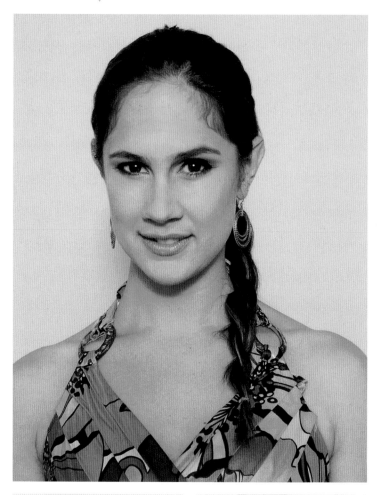

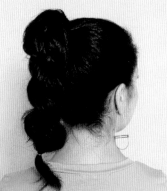

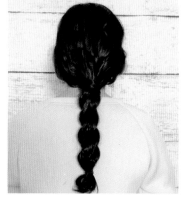

HOW TO DO IT

WHAT YOU NEED

- Hair serum
- Comb
- Hair ties

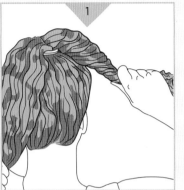

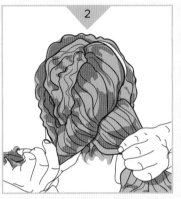

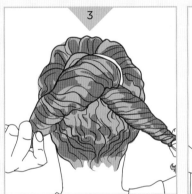

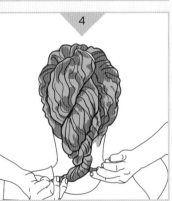

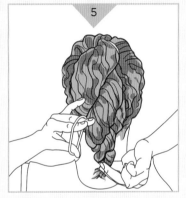

1. Apply some serum first to take care of any frizz. This style focuses on definition, so you want your curls to lay smooth. Comb your hair into a high ponytail and secure it with a hair tie, then divide this in two. Begin twisting the strand on your right side, in a clockwise direction.

2. Next, pass the right twist up and over the left section. Your left section should now be on the right.

3. Take the section that is now on your right side and begin twisting it clockwise, as before.

4. Lift this section up and over to the left. Then continue with this process, lifting right over left repeatedly until you reach the end of your hair.

5. Secure the end of the rope ponytail with a hair tie.

TOP TIP

Although this is a simple, casual look, you can always use an extra dose of serum to smooth down any stray hairs along your hairline to keep things looking extra clean and defined.

CURLY PUFF PONYTAIL

BEST FOR
Short to medium-length hair

ACCESSORIES
Accessorize this style with decorative bobby pins placed across the crown, or add a vibrant headband.

DIFFICULTY LEVEL
Easy

ASSISTANCE NEEDED?
No

Curly girls rule the puff ponytail. This 1970s-inspired 'do has made a comeback, which is good news for all of us, especially considering how quick it is to pull this one off! This is a more coiffed version of your curly ponytail, and it's a great style to choose for unwashed three-day hair. Just make sure you smooth your hairline with a curl definer to keep everything looking slick.

TRY THIS
Concentrate on contouring cheeks and eyes with a matte bronzer and eyeshadow. This will keep the look classy and simple.

SEE ALSO
High ponytail, pages 58–59
Pompadour ponytail, pages 88–89

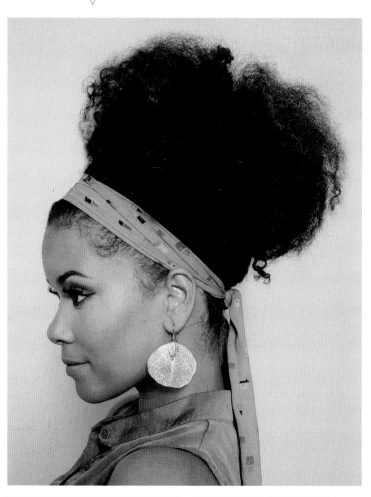

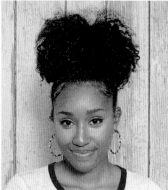

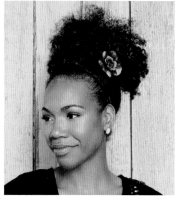

HOW TO DO IT

WHAT YOU NEED

- Curl definer
- Hairbrush or comb
- Hair tie
- Bobby pins
- Hair pick (optional)

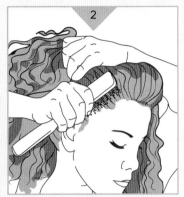

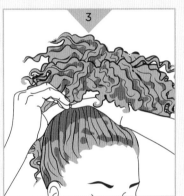

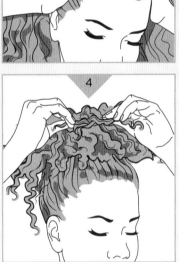

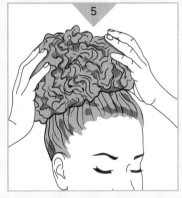

1. Start with three-day hair for the best results, and begin by massaging some curl definer along your hairline.

2. Use a thick hairbrush or comb to make the edges of your hair even smoother.

3. Gather up your hair into a high ponytail. Wrap the hair tie around your ponytail a few times, making sure it feels secure.

4. Use your fingers to separate your curls. Frizz is your friend with this 'do, so lift and separate each curl.

5. To finish off, create a rounded effect by molding your puff with the palms of your hands. If you have sufficient curl the puff should remain in place, although a few well-placed bobby pins will help to create the shape you desire if you have looser curls.

TOP TIP

Spritz a little water onto your hands and massage it into the puff to promote a more frizzy, coiffed puff. You can also create a bit of extra volume by working gently at the base of the ponytail with a hair pick.

DOUBLE-TWIST SIDE PONYTAIL

BEST FOR
Long hair

ACCESSORIES
To make this style really pop, slide a few decorative bobby pins into the completed twists.

DIFFICULTY LEVEL
Hard

ASSISTANCE NEEDED?
No

This topsy-turvy pony is a great way to switch up your everyday low pony, and the inside-out twist design looks gorgeous on any hair type. It's an elegant style that works well for date nights and other special occasions, but it's soft and pretty (and easy) enough for school or office, too!

TRY THIS
If you have shorter hair, you can adapt this style by parting your hair in half horizontally first, creating a half-up half-down version. Whatever your hair length, you can also leave strands of hair hanging loose in front of your ears to display your curls to best effect.

SEE ALSO
Two-twist low ponytail, pages 70–71
Side bun with twisted bangs, pages 128–29

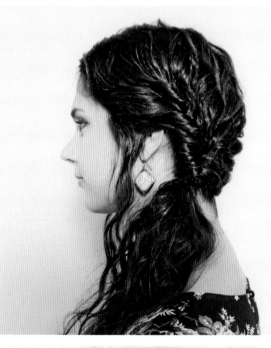

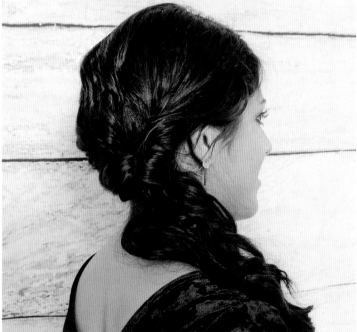

HOW TO DO IT

WHAT YOU NEED

- Hair tie
- Bobby pins

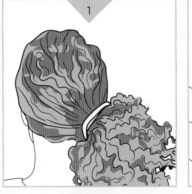

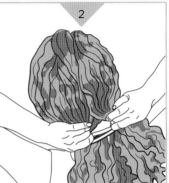

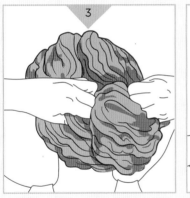

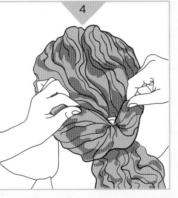

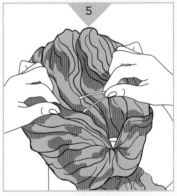

1. Gather all of your hair toward the lower right (or left) side of your head and secure it in a ponytail.

2. With both hands, create a gap right at the top of the ponytail, in the middle, just above your hair tie.

3. Now lift the ends of your ponytail and pass them through this gap—pull them all the way through to create the topsy-turvy effect. If you find this tricky, try holding the gap open with one hand while you use the other to pull the ponytail through.

4. Once it is all the way through, lift the raised sides of the ponytail slightly to exaggerate the look.

5. As you lift each side, slide a few bobby pins inside it to hold things in place. As you adjust the sides, you can also arrange the hair so that the hair tie is concealed.

TOP TIP

If you want to create this style on wet hair, use the two-strand twist-out method first (pages 48–49) and leave the twists in for 20 to 30 minutes to enhance your curl pattern before you begin styling.

TWISTED HALF-UP PONYTAIL

BEST FOR
Medium to long hair

ACCESSORIES
Dangly earrings and a few thin bangles are a cute combo for this style.

DIFFICULTY LEVEL
Medium

ASSISTANCE NEEDED?
No

I love the way that two simple twists can add so much dimension to curly hair. These chunky twists are pretty enough to wear on any occasion and, with just a bit of practice, they are very easy to create. This style can be worn on wet or dry hair.

TRY THIS
This is an ultra feminine hairstyle, so why not try bold lashes, contoured eyes, and a matte color on your lips? You can also opt to wear the remainder of your hair in a ponytail if you don't fancy this half-up half-down version.

SEE ALSO
Two-twist low ponytail, pages 70–71
Double-twist side ponytail, pages 76–77

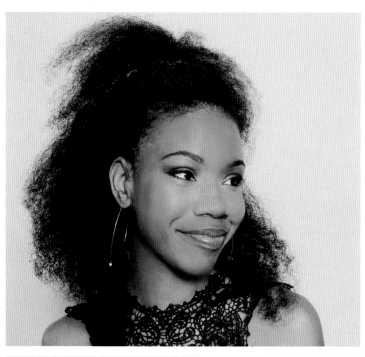

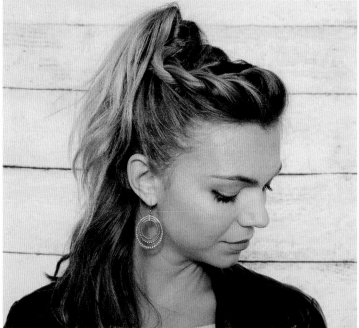

HOW TO DO IT

WHAT YOU NEED

- Comb
- Hair ties
- Bobby pins
- Curl definer (optional)

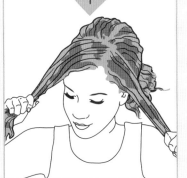

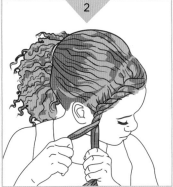

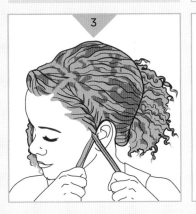

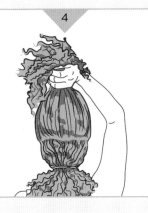

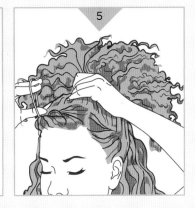

1. Create a part running from the front of one ear across to the other. Tie the rest of your hair out of the way for now, then create a side part in the upper section.

2. Working with one of the two front sections you've just created, begin flat-twisting your hair toward your ear, using the instructions on page 50. Twist until you reach your ear and then hold the twist in place with a few bobby pins.

3. Now repeat the flat-twisting process on the other side.

4. Release the remainder of your hair and use a comb to divide it in half horizontally.

5. Leave the lower section hanging free, but gather the top section, along with the twists, into a high ponytail. Once your hair tie is secure, loosen your ponytail a bit if you need to create extra fullness around your crown.

TOP TIP

For best results, start with wet hair. Apply some curl definer, then flip your head over and blow-dry your hair using a diffuser attachment, scrunching your hair as you work. This will create extra bounce and volume before you start styling.

LOW PONYTAIL
WITH MIDDLE PART

BEST FOR
Medium to long hair

ACCESSORIES
Make the most of the fact that your hair will be pulled back away from your face by wearing your favorite earrings.

DIFFICULTY LEVEL
Easy

ASSISTANCE NEEDED?
No

A middle part pairs very well with curly hair and gives an extra edge to the regular low ponytail with very little extra effort. The part also gives this style a polished and professional look, although it can work just as well for more casual occasions. It looks great worn wet or dry, too.

TRY THIS
A very simple variation on this style is to wear your ponytail to the side, like the low curly side ponytail shown on page 56. You can also wrap a strand of hair around your hair tie for an easy finishing touch.

SEE ALSO
Low curly side ponytail, pages 56–57
Wrapped ponytail, pages 64–65

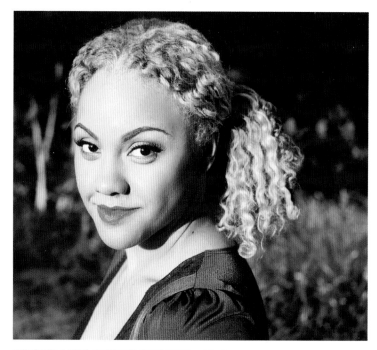

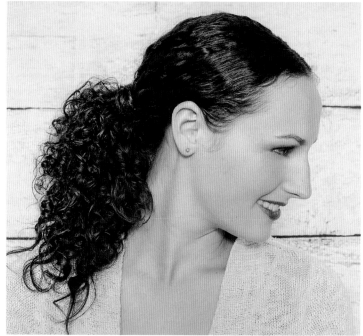

HOW TO DO IT

WHAT YOU NEED

- Comb
- Hair tie
- Bobby pins
- Hairspray
- Curl definer (optional)

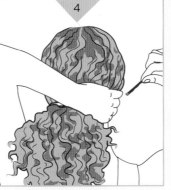

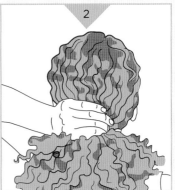

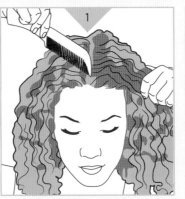

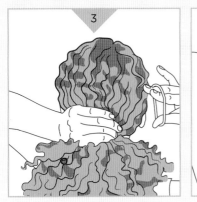

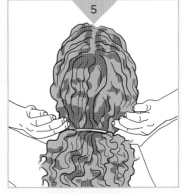

1. Begin by using a comb to create a neat middle part, running from your hairline to the crown of your head.

2. Now smooth your hair toward the back of your head, taking care to retain the middle part you just created.

3. Gather your hair into a low ponytail and secure it with a hair tie.

4. Once your ponytail is in position, smooth away any stray hairs and loose strands with your fingers and pin them out of the way, positioning the bobby pins behind your ears so that they are not visible.

5. Complete the look by grabbing your hair just above the hair tie. Carefully pull it outward to create a fuller appearance, then set everything with hairspray.

TOP TIP

If you want to create a slicker, more polished look, use a curl definer designed for curly hair to smooth down any stray strands of hair before pinning them behind your ears.

LOW PONYTAIL WITH SIDE BANGS

BEST FOR
All hair lengths

ACCESSORIES
The simplest and most effective way to dress up this hairstyle is by adding a bold, colorful headband.

DIFFICULTY LEVEL
Easy

ASSISTANCE NEEDED
No

Bangs are a great way to take a simple hairstyle and make it really pop, your ponytail and bangs providing two different focal points. Side bangs also bring attention to your face by framing it, and they are a great way of showcasing curly hair, whether you have tight spirals or gentle waves. This style is best worn with dry hair.

TRY THIS
Since the bangs focus attention on the center of your face, it makes sense to take your makeup up a notch, too. Apply both mascara and eyeliner for lots of definition around the eyes, then finish with your favorite lip color.

▶ **SEE ALSO**
Low curly side ponytail, pages 56–57
Low ponytail with middle part, pages 80–81

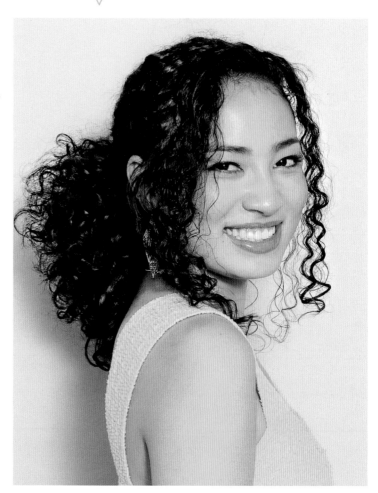

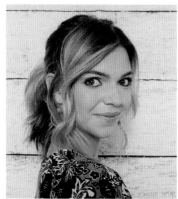

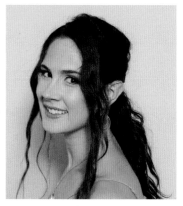

HOW TO DO IT

WHAT YOU NEED

- Comb
- Curl definer
- Hair tie
- Bobby pins
- Hairspray

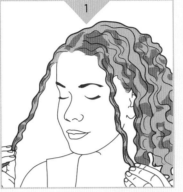

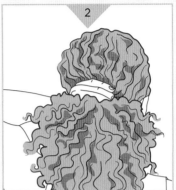

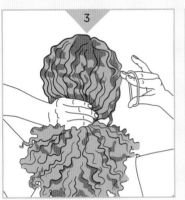

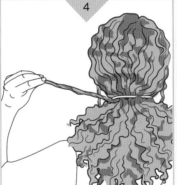

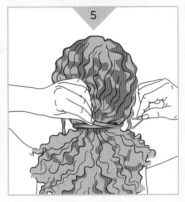

1. Take two small equal-sized strands of hair at the forehead, one from each side of your head, and separate them from the rest of your hair, using a comb. Massage these strands with a small amount of curl definer to create a bit of definition—particularly important if your hair is prone to frizziness.

2. Now gather the rest of your hair into a low ponytail. If you like, you can finger through your curls with a little more curl definer to create a smoother finish.

3. Secure the ponytail in place with a hair tie.

4. Take hold of a small strand of hair from your ponytail.

5. Wrap this strand around the hair tie, pinning the end into the base of the ponytail. When you are done you can neaten the whole look by securing any stray hairs with pins, and then setting everything with hairspray.

TOP TIP

This style can be easily modified into the high-crown ponytail (page 62), while keeping the bangs in place. If you have shorter hair, you can gently tug the hair at the back of your ponytail to create the illusion of extra length.

HIGH PONYTAIL WITH SIDE BRAID

BEST FOR
Medium to long hair

ACCESSORIES
Jewelry is the best option here, as you don't want to take away from the main focus of the style—the braid—by introducing hair accessories. Love street style? Then add some hoops to glam up this 'do.

DIFFICULTY LEVEL
Medium

ASSISTANCE NEEDED?
No

Sometimes every girl needs some hairspiration! Give your standard ponytail a much-needed revamp by adding in a thick, Dutch side braid—you'll be surprised by how this simple accent creates an entirely different feel. This look is chic and simple, and provides a quick add-on in the morning when you're looking for a perfect last-minute style.

TRY THIS
Gently use your fingers to lift the strands of the braid without unraveling it. This will widen the braid and give it a bolder look.

SEE ALSO
High bun with crown braid, pages 126–27
Double side braids, pages 144–45

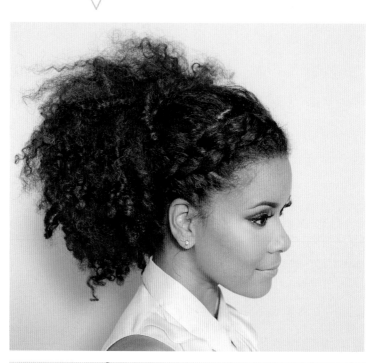

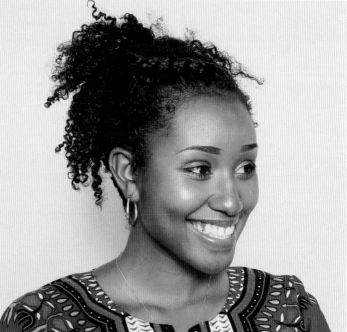

HOW TO DO IT

WHAT YOU NEED

- Comb
- Hair tie
- Bobby pins

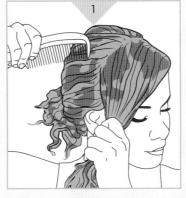

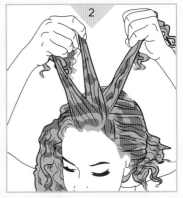

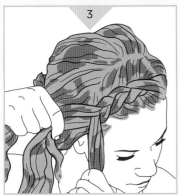

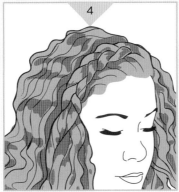

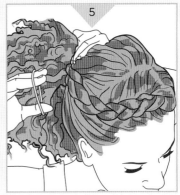

1. Use a comb to separate out a square section of hair along your forehead. This will be your braid. Put the rest of your hair in a low ponytail for now to keep it out of the way while you work.

2. Separate out three equal strands of hair from the start of your top section.

3. Begin Dutch braiding this section, following the instructions on page 149. Work across to the end part, staying parallel with your hairline, incorporating hair from either side of the braid as you work. When you reach the other part, continue to braid the hair for a little longer—or all the way to the ends if you prefer. Secure the end of the braid with a tie or pin for now.

4. Now release the rest of your hair from its ponytail.

5. Sweep all of your hair up into a high ponytail, incorporating your braid, then secure everything with a hair tie.

TOP TIP

The best way to keep bobby pins hidden is to slide them underneath your hair. Instead of widening the opening of the pin before inserting it, simply slide the closed pin into place and it will hold your hair perfectly.

HALF-UP HALF-DOWN PONYTAIL

BEST FOR
Medium to long hair

ACCESSORIES
Play up this fun hairstyle with some long, dangly earrings and a cute headband.

DIFFICULTY LEVEL
Easy

ASSISTANCE NEEDED?
No

This is a super cute hairstyle, and yet its chic simplicity means that it can also be adopted for more formal occasions. It's best styled on dry hair, and it will work with all hair types. Its other advantage is that it highlights your features by being drawn back from your forehead, while also framing your face lower down with the fullness retained to either side.

TRY THIS
This style is perfect for the basic ponytail kind of girl who likes to wear her hair down but away from her face. Eyeliner and a little lip gloss are all you need to make the most of this style.

SEE ALSO
High-crown ponytail, pages 62–63
High ponytail with rolled bangs, pages 90–91

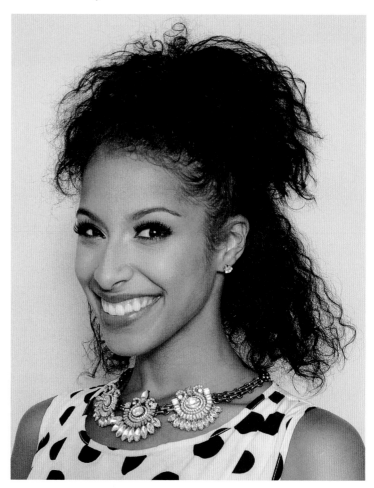

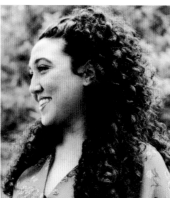

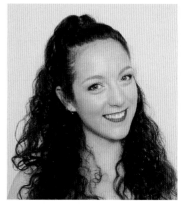

HOW TO DO IT

WHAT YOU NEED

- Comb
- Hair tie
- Hairspray
- Bobby pins
- Curl definer (optional)

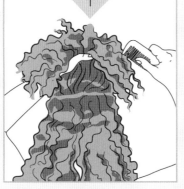

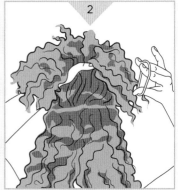

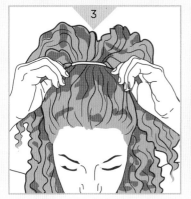

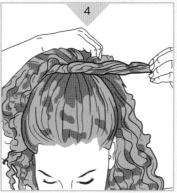

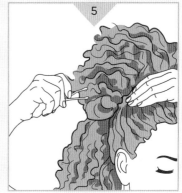

1. Start by using your comb to section your hair in half horizontally across the crown.

2. Now secure the upper section of hair with a hair tie to form your top ponytail.

3. Grab the hair at the base of your ponytail, where it meets the hair tie, and loosen it a bit so that the ponytail is not too tight. This will create more shape around your head.

4. Smooth any stray hairs with your fingers and use hairspray to help keep them in place throughout the day. Then, to give this familiar style a bit of a twist, take a small strand of hair from your ponytail and wrap it around the hair tie.

5. Secure the end of the strand in place with a few bobby pins.

TOP TIP

For a more polished look, concentrate on smoothing down any small stray hairs left along your hairline with the help of some curl definer.

POMPADOUR PONYTAIL

BEST FOR
Medium to long hair

ACCESSORIES
A patterned scarf goes very well with this hairstyle. Try polka dots or an animal print to play up your look even more. Small hoop earrings are another great match for this saucy look.

DIFFICULTY LEVEL
Medium

ASSISTANCE NEEDED?
No

Want to jazz up your ponytail? This hairstyle takes the humble side pony to the next level by adding a pompadour, creating a retro style that's perfect for curlies who want an edgier look. The pompadour also takes advantage of the fact that it can be much easier to keep curly hair in place than straight hair!

TRY THIS
The tutorial on the opposite page demonstrates this style with a low side ponytail, but you can play with the position of the pony, as seen in the photos here.

SEE ALSO
Low curly side ponytail, pages 56–57
High ponytail with rolled bangs, pages 90–91

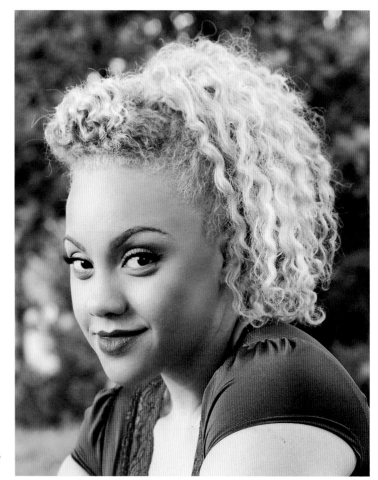

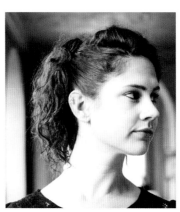

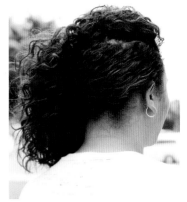

HOW TO DO IT

WHAT YOU NEED

- Curl definer
- Comb
- Bobby pins
- Hair tie
- Hairspray

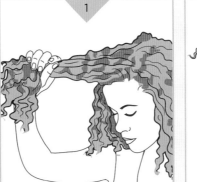

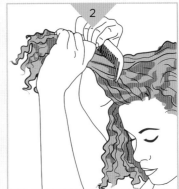

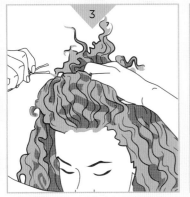

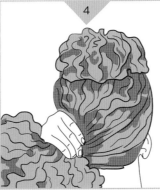

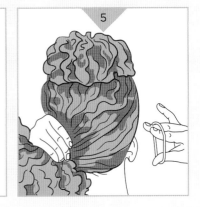

1. Apply a small amount of curl definer to begin, then separate out a square section at the front of your head. This will form your pompadour.

2. Backcomb this top section of hair to create some volume.

3. When you have created sufficient volume, lift this section while also pushing it forward so that it forms a soft peak, then secure it with plenty of bobby pins.

4. The rest of your hair can now be gathered together into a low side ponytail, making sure you don't disturb the pompadour. Use your hands or the comb to keep everything looking nice and smooth.

5. Finish off by securing the ponytail with a hair tie, and then set everything in place with some hairspray.

TOP TIP

Providing your pompadour with sufficient hold is essential to keeping this look intact throughout the day, so don't be tempted to skip the backcombing or the hairspray!

HIGH PONYTAIL
WITH ROLLED BANGS

BEST FOR
All hair lengths

ACCESSORIES
A patterned headband or headscarf would be the ideal vintage-style addition here.

DIFFICULTY LEVEL
Medium

ASSISTANCE NEEDED?
No

Who doesn't love vintage hair? This pinup-inspired 'do has a classic feel, and it also manages to be both easy and edgy. The rolled bangs are a quick touch that really help bring the whole look to life. This style looks great on all curl types, from the loosest wave to the tightest coil. And let's be honest—every girl should have at least one vintage-inspired style in her collection!

TRY THIS
A bright red or burgundy lip and winged liner combo are ideal with this hairstyle.

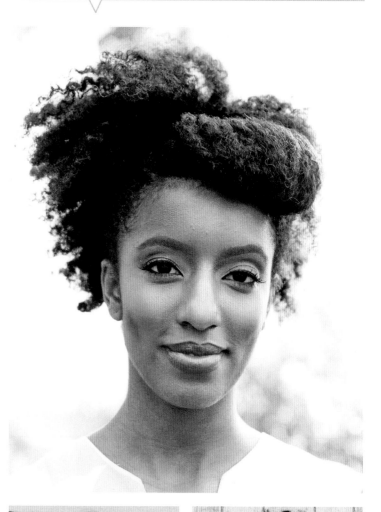

▶ **SEE ALSO**
Victory rolls, pages 116–17
Low bun with rolled bangs, pages 118–19

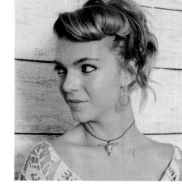

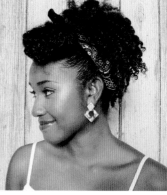

HOW TO DO IT

WHAT YOU NEED

- Bobby pins
- Hair tie
- Hairbrush
- Curl definer
- Hairspray (optional)

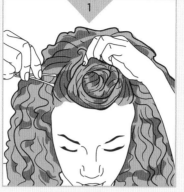

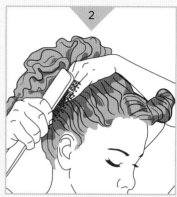

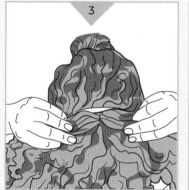

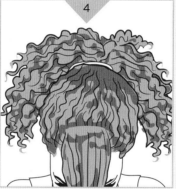

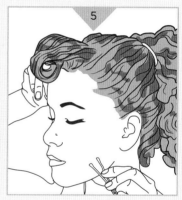

1. Separate out a small, square section at your forehead for the bangs. Use bobby pins to keep it separate from the rest of your hair for now.

2. Gather the rest of your hair up into a high ponytail, securing it with a hair tie. Use a brush and some curl definer to smooth the hair around your hairline, to keep the pony looking neat and polished.

3. Tighten the ponytail a little bit by grabbing the hair close to the band and gently tugging it in opposite directions. Be careful not to dislodge the position of the ponytail, though.

4. Now remove the bobby pins from your bangs.

5. Use your pointer finger and middle finger on each hand to roll your bangs up and under toward your scalp, then slide a few bobby pins underneath carefully to hold them in place.

TOP TIP

If you have a finer curl type and you have problems keeping the bangs in place, lightly spritz them with hairspray for extra hold.

BUBBLE PONYTAIL

BEST FOR

Long hair

ACCESSORIES

Adding multicolored mini hair ties between each bubble creates a fun, vibrant effect.

DIFFICULTY LEVEL

Easy

ASSISTANCE NEEDED?

No

I adore this creative twist on the everyday ponytail. It's a quick option for when you're pressed for time, but the bubble effect gives it so much character that it can serve you well for special occasions, too. This style is perhaps best suited to looser curl types, although it's one that every curly should try!

TRY THIS

This pony looks good enough as it is, but try raising the hair at the crown, pompadour style, if you want to make it more dramatic. Simply backcomb it a little at the roots before forming your initial ponytail. You may also want to wrap a small strand of hair around each hair tie for extra polish.

SEE ALSO

Rope ponytail, pages 72–73
Triple crown twists,
pages 138–39

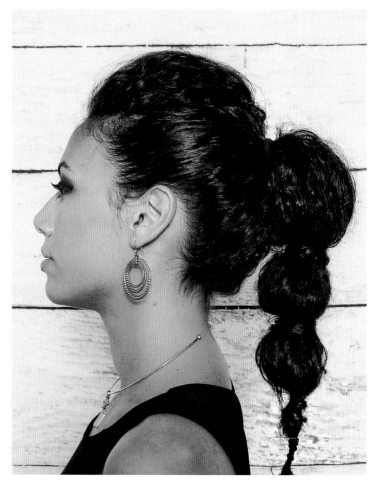

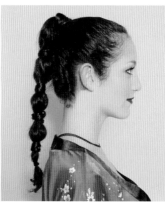

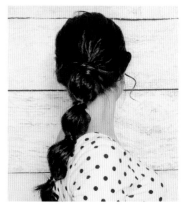

HOW TO DO IT

WHAT YOU NEED

- Hair ties
- Hair clip or pin
- Comb

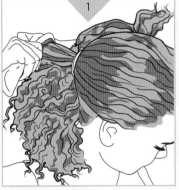

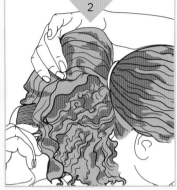

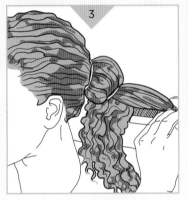

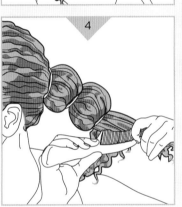

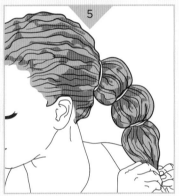

1. Gather your hair, bring it to the back of your head, and secure it with a hair tie. Separate out a small strand at the top of your ponytail, then use a hair clip or bobby pin to hold it up out of the way.

2. Now begin teasing the hair of the ponytail with a comb, just below the hair tie. When you have sufficient volume, free up the strand you separated earlier, and use your comb to gently smooth this hair over the teased section.

3. Use a hair tie to secure the ponytail just below this "bubble," a few inches away from the first hair tie.

4. Repeat Steps 1 to 3 to create a second bubble, and then a third, or continue until you reach the end of your hair.

5. Secure the end of the ponytail with a hair tie.

TOP TIP

Use some curl definer to smooth out each bubble. This will neaten the overall look and make each bubble more pronounced. You can also "fatten" the bubbles by pulling them outward gently with your fingers.

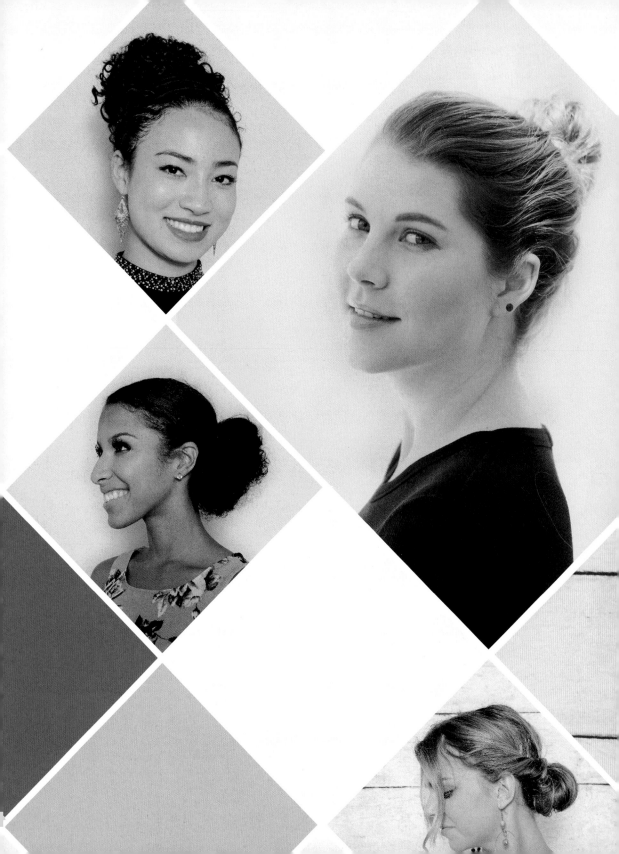

BUNS AND KNOTS

HALO BUN

BEST FOR
Medium to long hair

ACCESSORIES
The "halo" created by the three headbands used opposite gives this style plenty of interest, but you can always add earrings if you want to draw more attention to your features.

DIFFICULTY LEVEL
Easy

ASSISTANCE NEEDED?
No

Bored with the ordinary bun? Then try this classic, pretty style for a change. The "headbands" are actually just thin strips of fabric tied at the back. They are a simple touch that will give you a whole new look, and one that will really flatter your curly hair. I designed this 'do to create the illusion of fuller hair. It's simple, elegant, and suits all curls.

TRY THIS
Switch up the placement of the bun for a little variety. You can wear it high, to the side, or low.

SEE ALSO
High bun with swooped bangs, pages 102–03
Curly bun with faux bangs, pages 114–15

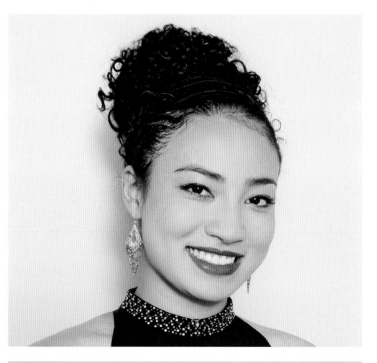

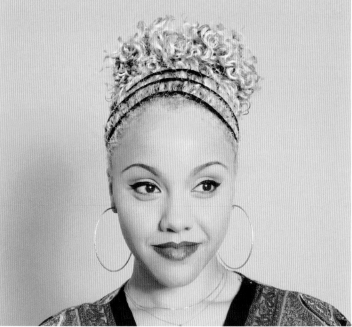

HOW TO DO IT

WHAT YOU NEED

- Comb
- Hair tie
- Bobby pins
- Hairspray
- Three thin strips of fabric, long enough to tie at the back

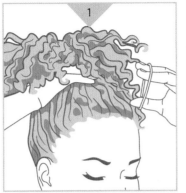

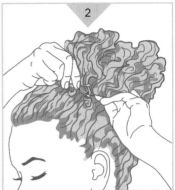

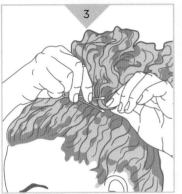

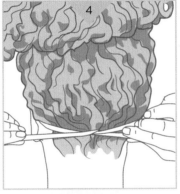

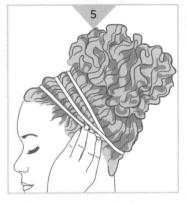

1. For this style, dry second- or third-day hair is ideal; your hair will have more volume. Gather it up into a high ponytail and secure it with a hair tie. (If you need extra volume, backcomb your pony before moving on to the next step.)

2. Gather and fold the ponytail under to create a bun, and use pins to hold it in place. Experiment with the pins to perfect the shape of your bun. Hairspray will help hold it in place, too.

3. For a polished look, do a quick check and secure any last stray strands of hair with a few more bobby pins.

4. Now tie the first "headband" around your head as shown, securing it at the back.

5. Add the other two bands in turn, leaving half an inch between each on top, but tapering them to overlap at the back.

TOP TIP

For an easy variation, try spacing the headbands even farther apart—about an inch. This will create the ultimate illusion of thicker hair.

HALO TWIST

BEST FOR
All hair lengths

ACCESSORIES
Decorative bobby pins are the perfect accessory for this 'do. Bring focus to your halo twist by sliding festive pins an inch apart along your hairline.

DIFFICULTY LEVEL
Easy

ASSISTANCE NEEDED?
No

The halo twist is an easy style for those of you who like to wear your hair down, but without the worry of having hair in your face. It's simple to create, and ideal for all curly and kinky types and textures. Second-day hair works best for this style, so you don't even need to worry about washing your hair!

TRY THIS
Add glamour to this look by wearing a bold smoky eye and soft lip and cheek color.

SEE ALSO
Side bun with twisted bangs, pages 128–29
Triple crown twists, pages 138–39

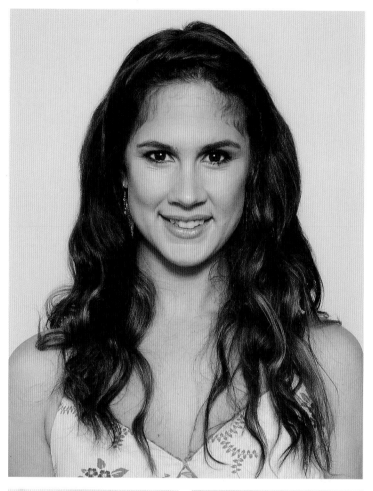

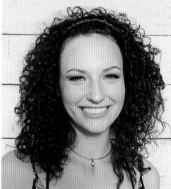

HOW TO DO IT

WHAT YOU NEED

- Comb
- Hair tie
- Curl definer
- Bobby pins

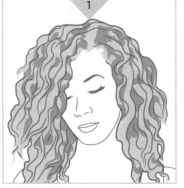

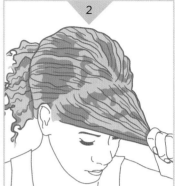

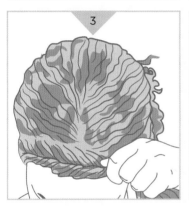

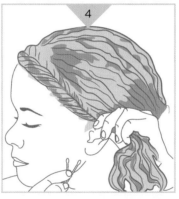

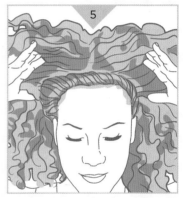

1. This hairstyle works best on curls that have volume, so second- or even third-day dry hair is ideal.

2. Part a small section from the front of one ear to the opposite side. Gather the rest of your hair into a low bun or ponytail.

3. Now begin twisting the small front section from one side towards the other, following the instructions on page 50. A bit of curl definer will give you a smoother, more finished look.

4. Once you've reached the opposite side of your head, secure the twist behind your ear with bobby pins.

5. Release the rest of your hair and run your fingers through your curls to plump them out and complete the look.

TOP TIP

Don't fret if your twist isn't perfect the first time. Because you're twisting across your hairline, it can be hard to see what you're doing. Stop when you're halfway across, check that the twist is looking neat, then continue on your way.

TWISTED CHIGNON

BEST FOR
Medium to long hair

ACCESSORIES
Bold accessories look great with this style. Try a chunky necklace or some large stud earrings. If you prefer less drama, smaller stud earrings look great also.

DIFFICULTY LEVEL
Medium

ASSISTANCE NEEDED?
No

The twisted chignon is simply gorgeous on any hair type. Though you can opt for this look whenever you like, I think a classic like this is best saved for special occasions, like a girls' night out or a date with your beau. This style really makes the most of your curls, showing off their texture to best effect.

TRY THIS
Want to add even more flair to this hairstyle? Double up on the twists to give it a whole new feel with very little extra effort.

SEE ALSO
Curly bun with faux bangs, pages 114–15
Messy French twist, pages 170–71

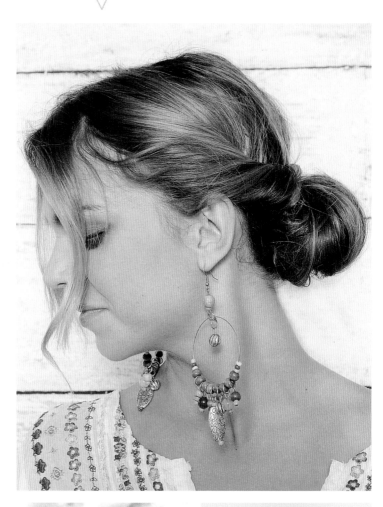

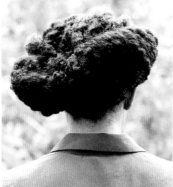

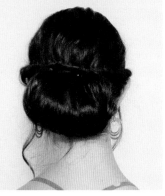

HOW TO DO IT

WHAT YOU NEED

- Comb
- Hair tie
- Bobby pins
- Hair donut (optional)

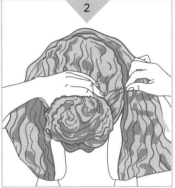

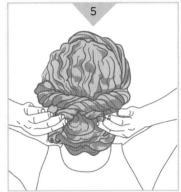

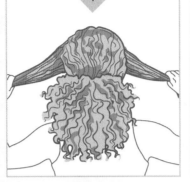

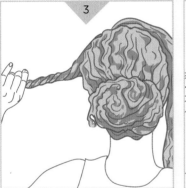

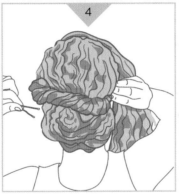

1. Separate out a small rectangular section along your hairline—the part should run from one ear to the other. Divide this section in half and slip the rest of your hair into a low ponytail.

2. Grab the ends of your ponytail and fold them up toward the hair tie. Secure the ends with a few bobby pins.

3. Take the left section and begin twisting it from root to tip.

4. Take this twist across the back of your head, over and round to the far side of your bun. This should conceal any straggly ends from your bun, too. Pin the end of the twist near the hair tie.

5. Now twist the section on your right side, then pass it over the previous twist and round to the opposite side of the bun, pinning in place as before. Finish off by pulling on both sides of the bun to loosen it and give it extra volume.

TOP TIP

If you have really fine hair, you can always cheat by wrapping it around a hair donut instead of creating the bun shown here!

HIGH BUN
WITH SWOOPED BANGS

BEST FOR
Medium to long hair

ACCESSORIES
Add flowers, a headscarf, or some hair jewelry to take this style to the next level.

DIFFICULTY LEVEL
Medium

ASSISTANCE NEEDED?
No

If you're a bun-and-bangs kind of girl, this might be just the hairstyle you're looking for. It's simple, fun, and chic. It's also very easy to create once you know what you're doing, and is the sort of 'do that adapts to almost any occasion—it's a real case of "one style fits all"! Just make sure everything is securely pinned and sprayed in place before you head out.

TRY THIS
Bangs bring so much attention to the center of your face. Celebrate this and accent your hairstyle with bold lashes and your favorite lip color.

▶ **SEE ALSO**
Low bun with swooped bangs, pages 112–13
High bun with crown braid, pages 126–27

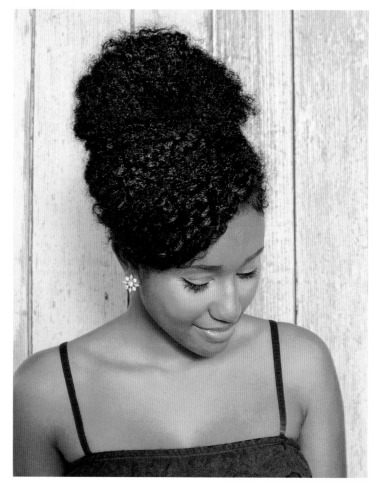

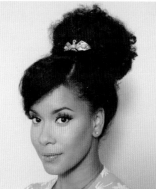

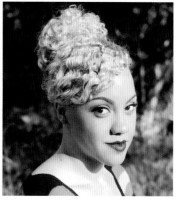

HOW TO DO IT

WHAT YOU NEED

- Comb
- Bobby pins
- Hair tie
- Hairspray (optional)

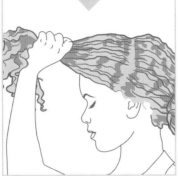

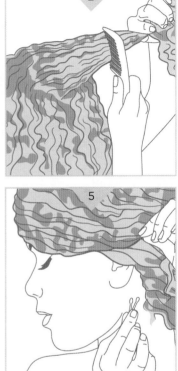

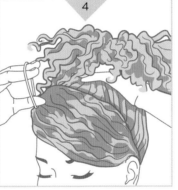

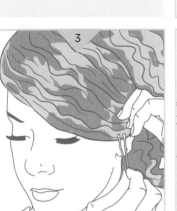

1. Use a comb to part off a section at your forehead. This will be your bangs. Tie the rest of your hair out of the way for now.

2. Lift a small piece of hair in the middle of this section and backcomb it to add a little volume.

3. Now sweep the bangs across your face and secure them behind your ear with a couple of bobby pins.

4. Lift the remainder of hair up toward your crown and secure it with a hair tie to form a high bun.

5. If you want a neater look, take care of any stray hairs by pinning them in place—with curly hair you have the advantage of being able to hide pins in your hair much more easily than with straight hair. Have at it!

TOP TIP

Even if you've used plenty of pins, you can also help make sure your style has all the staying power it will need by applying hairspray once you're done.

ROPE-BRAID BUN

BEST FOR
Long hair

ACCESSORIES
Decorative, glittery bobby pins or a bun cuff are great additions to this style.

DIFFICULTY LEVEL
Medium

ASSISTANCE NEEDED?
No

As any curly-haired girl knows, you can always add another bun to the mix! This bun is a twist—literally!—on the rope ponytail, and it's an easy and convenient style to choose when you want to step up your bun game. What I love most about this style is how cleverly and effectively it creates the illusion of thicker hair.

TRY THIS
Any makeup look will work well with this versatile style. Go completely neutral or go bold; a different approach will create a fresh vibe every time.

SEE ALSO
Rope ponytail, pages 72–73
Cinnamon roll braid, pages 162–63

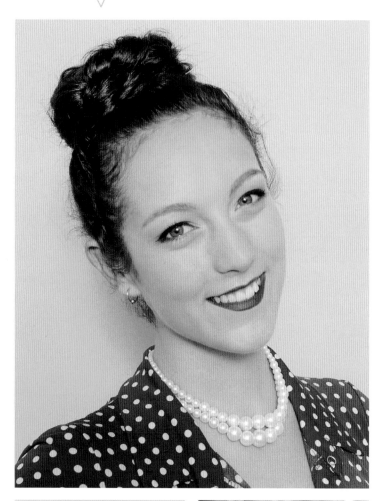

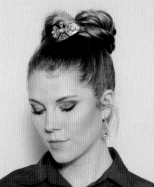

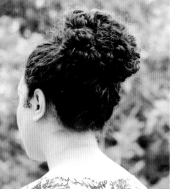

HOW TO DO IT

WHAT YOU NEED

- Hair ties
- Bobby pins

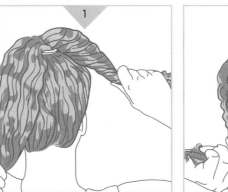

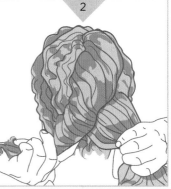

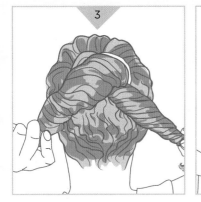

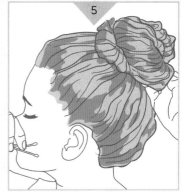

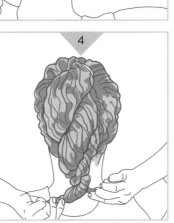

1. Gather your hair up into a high ponytail and secure with a hair tie, then divide it into two equal sections. Twist the section on your right, working in a clockwise direction.

2. Take this twisted section and pass it up and over the section on your left. The section that was on the left should now be on the right.

3. Now repeat the same process with the new right-hand section, twisting it clockwise and then passing it up and over.

4. Continue working this way down your ponytail, and then secure the finished rope braid with a hair tie.

5. Finally, create your bun by wrapping this rope braid around the base of your ponytail, using plenty of bobby pins to secure it.

TOP TIP

If you're feeling ambitious, why not try "accessorizing" this with some crown braids (see page 156) as an alternative to a regular headband?

FAUX CURLY BOB

BEST FOR
Medium to long hair

ACCESSORIES
Stud earrings really bring this
style to life, so break out the
pearls or diamonds!

DIFFICULTY LEVEL
Medium

ASSISTANCE NEEDED?
No

Long hair is great, but some
days you just fancy sporting
a shorter hairstyle for a change.
That's where the faux bob can
help! And, if you can create a
neat finish where the hair is
turned under, then it may even
pass for the real thing. Pins and
hairspray will help keep it intact,
but you will find it easiest to
work with second-day hair.

TRY THIS
One of the advantages of the
faux bob is that you can adjust
the part to your liking. For a
vintage feel, choose a middle
part. Or if you prefer bangs,
part your hair on one side,
sweep your bangs across your
face, then secure them with pins.

SEE ALSO
Twisted chignon, pages
100–01
Low twisted curls, pages
136–37

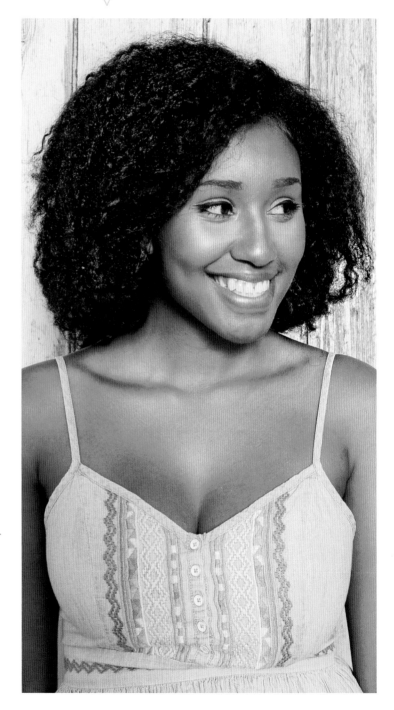

HOW TO DO IT

WHAT YOU NEED

- Comb
- Bobby pins
- Hairspray

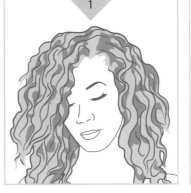

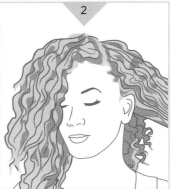

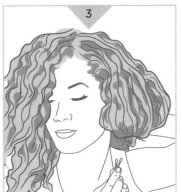

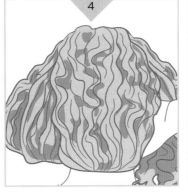

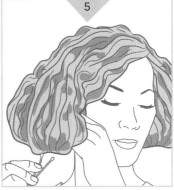

1. Start with dry, second-day hair—third-day hair can be even better. Hair that hasn't been washed for a day or two will give you much more volume to work with. Create a part on one side of your head, from the front of the hairline back to the crown.

2. Now separate out a large section of hair from one side.

3. Use your fingers to gently roll this section of hair under until it is the length that you would like. When the hair is sitting smoothly and level, secure it from underneath with pins.

4. Repeat this at the back of your head.

5. Complete the bob by rolling and pinning the hair on the other side of your head. If you have bangs you can tuck these in place now, securing them with pins. Finish with hairspray.

TOP TIP

For a consistent length all the way round, make sure you follow the procedure described here—pinning up one side first to establish the length, then completing the back and opposite side to match.

MESSY BUN

BEST FOR

Medium to long hair

ACCESSORIES

A messy bun looks great on its own, but it can instantly be taken up a notch by adding a colorful wide headband or a pair of hoop earrings.

DIFFICULTY LEVEL

Easy

ASSISTANCE NEEDED?

No

Whether you are off to the gym or heading out for a night on the town, the messy bun adds a little zest to the ordinary bun. The goal is to keep the hair around your bun looking sleek and soft, so use a curl definer if you need to. You can also play around with the bun to create the shape you prefer.

TRY THIS

For an even more casual look, a half-up half-down variation is a great choice. Both styles are simple, though, so you can play them up or down with makeup. Go bold on brows and lips, or keep everything neutral with a touch of mascara and lip gloss.

SEE ALSO

Halo bun, pages 96–97
Topknot, pages 120–21

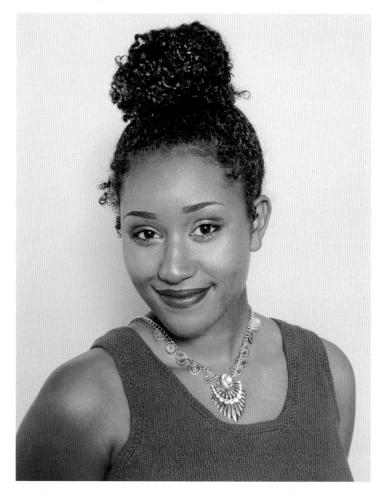

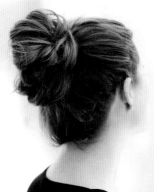

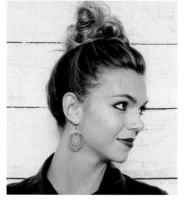

HOW TO DO IT

WHAT YOU NEED

- Curl definer
- Hair ties
- Comb
- Bobby pins

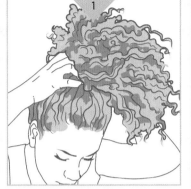
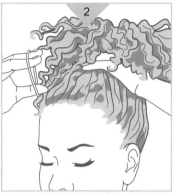
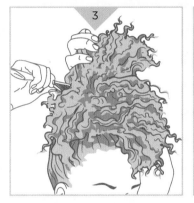
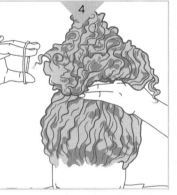
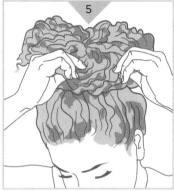

1. Second- or third-day hair is ideal for this style, since it will have a bit more body and natural hold. Starting with dry hair is key when creating a messy bun. You can also apply some curl definer at this stage. Begin by flipping your hair up and forward.

2. Use a tie to secure your hair at the crown in a high ponytail.

3. Now use your comb to thoroughly tease the hair around the base of your ponytail.

4. When you have created enough volume, gather your hair into a messy bun and secure it with a second hair tie.

5. Finally, use your fingers to loosen the bun. Experiment with the shape until you have something that looks right, and finish by pinning any stray hairs in place.

TOP TIP

If you have fine hair, make sure you backcomb as much as you need to so that your finished bun will have the fullness it needs for a messy effect.

LOW SIDE BUN

BEST FOR
Medium to long hair

ACCESSORIES
The simplest way to dress up this style is by adding in a bun clip at the base.

DIFFICULTY LEVEL
Easy

ASSISTANCE NEEDED?
No

The great thing about curly hair is that it makes the most of even very simple styles. The side bun is a great example of this. It is easy to create, and it will really accentuate your curls. This style can be worn either wet or dry, but if you have finer curls and want more volume, you will find that second-day hair works more effectively. If you want to give it even more life, try backcombing before you start.

TRY THIS
Adding a center or side part is a great way to change up this style. See the low ponytail with middle part on page 80.

▶ **SEE ALSO**
Rope-braid bun, pages 104–105
Low bun with rolled bangs, pages 118–19

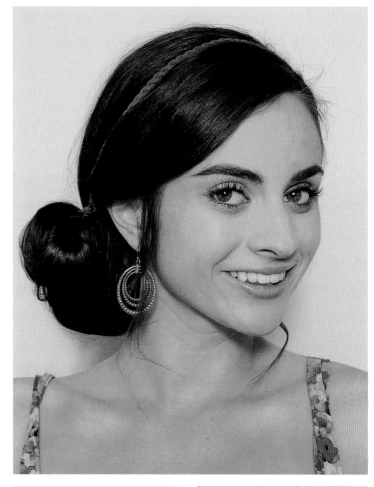

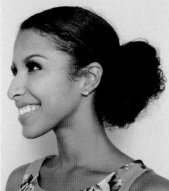

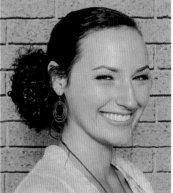

HOW TO DO IT

WHAT YOU NEED

- Curl definer
- Hair ties
- Bobby pins
- Hairspray
- Hair donut (optional)

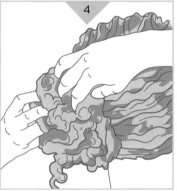

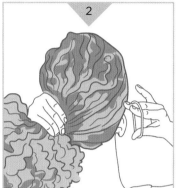

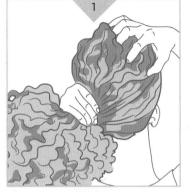

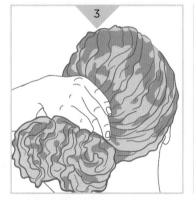

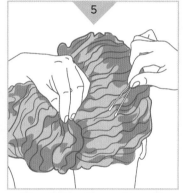

1. Use your fingers to smooth your hair toward the back of your head, and slightly to the side. You can smooth on a bit of curl definer at this point, too, if your hair needs it.

2. Use a hair tie to secure your hair into a low ponytail.

3. Now gather your ponytail into a bun and secure this with another hair tie.

4. Use your fingers to loosen the bun a bit, taking care not to dislodge the hair tie. This will give the bun more volume, and create the appearance of it sitting higher up on your head.

5. If there are any stray hairs after this, tuck them in with a few pins, and add a touch more curl definer along the hairline to create a sleeker look. Apply hairspray to finish if you want the style to be extra long-lasting.

TOP TIP

To create the illusion of a fuller bun, try using a hair donut instead of forming a natural bun. You could even try making your own custom-sized donut from an old sock—you'll find plenty of tutorials online for how to do this!

LOW BUN WITH SWOOPED BANGS

BEST FOR
Medium to long hair

ACCESSORIES
Take this style and make it red-carpet–worthy by wearing a statement necklace or some dangly earrings.

DIFFICULTY LEVEL
Medium

ASSISTANCE NEEDED?
No

This look is similar to the high bun with swooped bangs on page 102, but it has a more understated, professional look which is ideal for school, work, or more formal occasions. It's easy to achieve, too, so definitely one to add to your go-to list.

TRY THIS
As with most buns, you can rearrange the placement of this to create subtly different effects. Try it off to one side, as with the low side bun on page 110, or worn right down low, at the nape. You can also play with the placement of your bangs.

▶ **SEE ALSO**
High bun with swooped bangs, pages 102–03
Rope-braid bun, pages 104–05

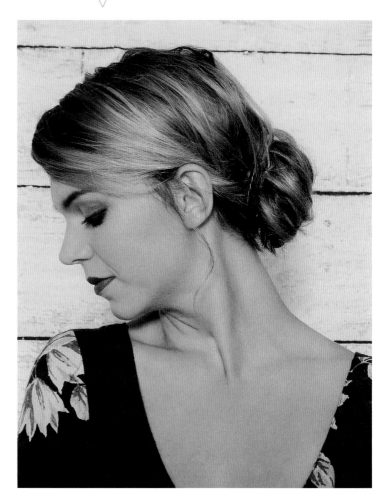

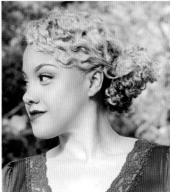

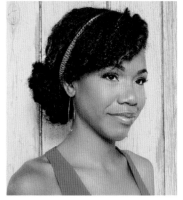

HOW TO DO IT

WHAT YOU NEED

- Comb
- Hair ties
- Curl definer
- Bobby pins
- Hairspray

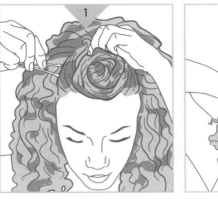

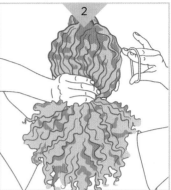

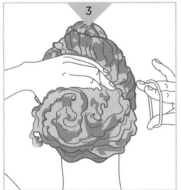

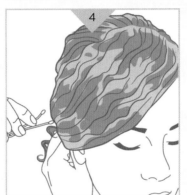

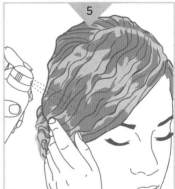

1. Separate out a small section of hair at your forehead to form your bangs, but pin this out of the way for now.

2. Use a hair tie to secure the rest of your hair into a low ponytail. A little curl definer applied to the sides of your head will help to smooth any stray hairs.

3. Gather up your ponytail and tuck it into a bun, securing it with another hair tie.

4. Now unpin your bangs and sweep them across your face, pinning the ends behind your ear.

5. Check for any last stray hairs, which can be pinned discretely in place, then finish off with an allover application of hairspray.

TOP TIP

If you want to add more volume to this style, backcomb your ponytail before creating the bun, and do the same with your bangs before draping them across your face. Make sure you spritz with plenty of hairspray to preserve the look.

CURLY BUN WITH FAUX BANGS

BEST FOR
Medium to long hair

ACCESSORIES
This style looks great all on its own, but if you want to make more of an impact, add a headband and a pair of dangly earrings.

DIFFICULTY LEVEL
Medium

ASSISTANCE NEEDED?
No

So you want bangs but you're not quite ready to chop off your hair? Introduce faux bangs into your life instead! Curly bangs can be hard to manage, and they tend to gravitate toward frizz, which can be a real pain. The great thing about faux bangs is that bobby pins keep them sitting nice and flat on your forehead. Experiment with this look on both wet and dry hair to see which you prefer.

TRY THIS
A half-up half-down version is an easy alternative to the look shown here. Just let the back portion of your hair hang freely.

▶ **SEE ALSO**
Low side bun, pages 110–11
High bun with crown braid, pages 126–27

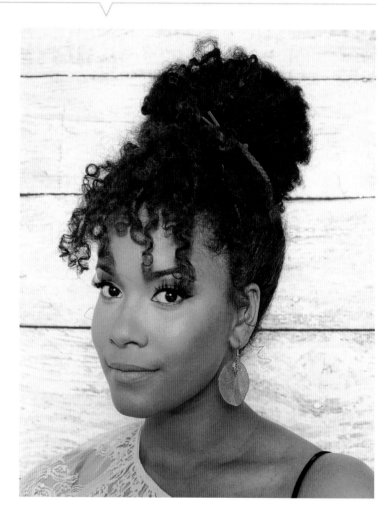

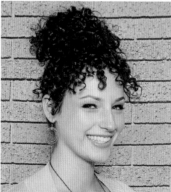

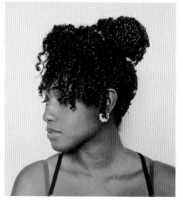

HOW TO DO IT

WHAT YOU NEED

- Hair tie
- Bobby pins
- Curl definer
- Foaming mousse (optional)

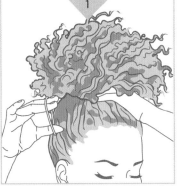

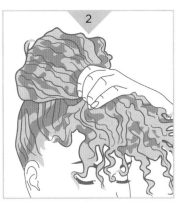

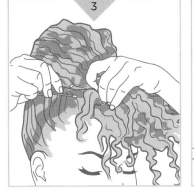

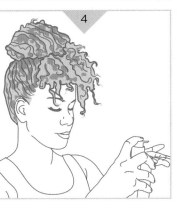

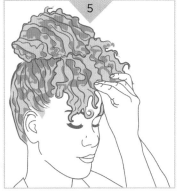

1. Gather all of your hair and lift it toward your crown, then secure it firmly into a high ponytail.

2. Bring the hair from your ponytail forward.

3. Now, holding your hair in place with one hand, use your free hand to begin sliding pins along the upturned portion of ponytail to create your faux bangs.

4. Pump out a dime-sized amount of curl definer and rub it between your fingers.

5. Apply the product to your curls to tame any frizz. Use your fingertips to work the product in gently, taking care not to dislodge your carefully created new bangs!

TOP TIP

If you're creating this style with wet hair, you can substitute foaming mousse for curl definer—this will help your curls maintain their definition throughout the day.

VICTORY ROLLS

BEST FOR
Medium to long hair

ACCESSORIES
Vintage styles call for accessories that recall the past! Tuck a flower behind your ear for the ultimate pinup girl look, or use a headscarf to bring focus to the rolls.

DIFFICULTY LEVEL
Medium/hard

ASSISTANCE NEEDED?
No

If you have a love for retro, this style will be right up your alley. It may take a bit of practice to get the rolls looking perfect, but once you've mastered them you will have a style that is ideal for special occasions, such as date nights and weddings. Dress it up with matching retro makeup or fun and flirty accessories. This style works best on dry hair.

TRY THIS
Although the tutorial opposite demonstrates how to create twin rolls, a single roll can be just as effective—and of course twice as fast!

SEE ALSO
Pompadour ponytail, pages 88–89
Twisted chignon, pages 100–01

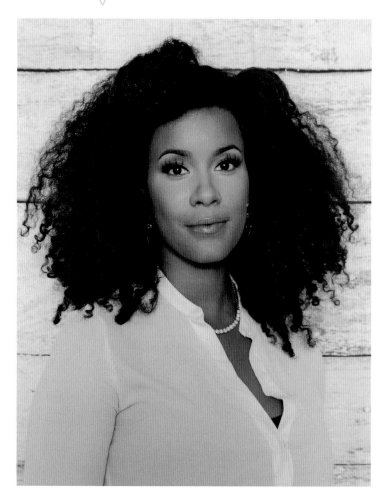

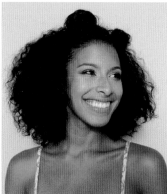

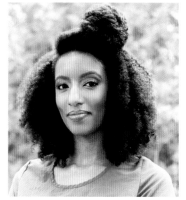

HOW TO DO IT

WHAT YOU NEED

- Curl definer
- Comb
- Bobby pins
- Hairspray

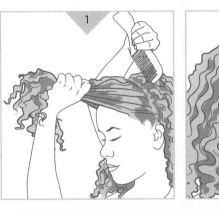

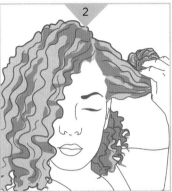

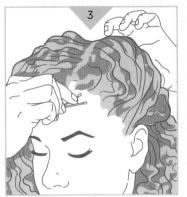

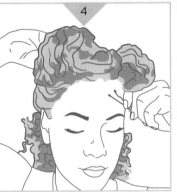

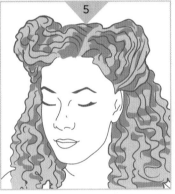

1. Apply a bit of curl definer to your hair, then using a comb separate out a small section of hair on top of your head, running the part from just in front of one ear horizontally across to the same place by the opposite ear.

2. Divide this top section of hair into two equal halves, then use your fingers to roll one half-section up toward your scalp.

3. Secure this first roll with bobby pins. Use as many as you need to keep it secure, and distribute them evenly around the roll.

4. Now repeat Steps 2 and 3 on the other side, making sure the second roll matches the shape, size, and position of the first.

5. Fluff up your free-hanging curls at the back and set with hairspray. You got this!

TOP TIP

When creating victory rolls, it's easy to feel like you're not getting it right. After the first few pins, stop and check that you have the desired size. If the roll is too big, simple tweak a few strands and use some extra pins to keep them in place.

LOW BUN WITH ROLLED BANGS

BEST FOR
Medium to long hair

ACCESSORIES
Keep it simple, or throw on a bright headscarf to give your 'do some extra flair and individuality.

DIFFICULTY LEVEL
Medium

ASSISTANCE NEEDED?
No

This look is both retro and bold. For curlies who have a love of classic hairstyles, this is the perfect addition to your style collection. It takes very little time in the morning to whip this one up once you've mastered the technique, and it works on wet or dry hair, and all textures and curl types.

TRY THIS
As you'd imagine, given its retro feel, this style pairs most effectively with a vintage-style bold lip or eye.

SEE ALSO
Halo bun, pages 96–97
Low bun with swooped bangs, pages 112–13

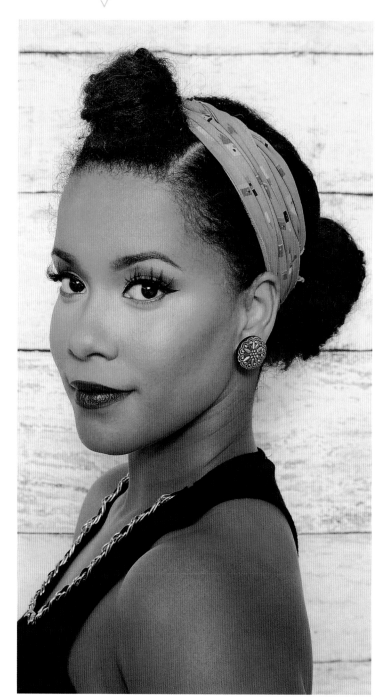

HOW TO DO IT

WHAT YOU NEED

- Curl definer
- Comb
- Bobby pins
- Hair ties
- Hairspray (optional)

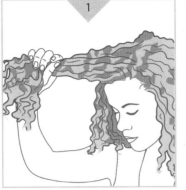

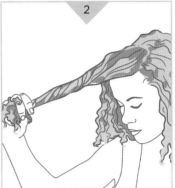

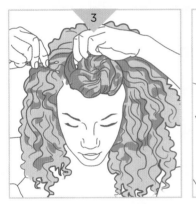

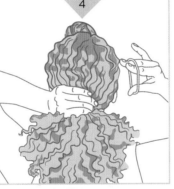

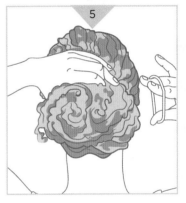

1. Begin by applying a small amount of curl definer to your hair, then using a comb, separate out a small section of hair on top. This is what you will use to create your bangs.

2. Holding this section out in front of you, twist it from root to tail.

3. Now carefully roll up the twisted section of hair with your fingers, working it into a spiral that sits against the top of your head. Secure the coil with enough pins to hold it in place.

4. Smooth the rest of your hair into a low ponytail and secure it with a hair tie.

5. Finish by gathering your ponytail up into a low bun and secure it with a second hair tie.

TOP TIP

You can adjust the shape of both the rolled bangs and the bun by using your fingers to loosen them once they have been rolled into place. Set them with hairspray to give them a bit of extra hold if you need to.

TOPKNOT

BEST FOR
All hair lengths

ACCESSORIES
Give this style a bohemian feel by wearing a pair of hoop earrings and a chunky bracelet or two.

DIFFICULTY LEVEL
Easy

ASSISTANCE NEEDED?
No

Lazy hair is the best hair! This style is the ultimate lazy 'do, and yet it still manages to be both chic and cute. A small top bun keeps your hair out of your eyes, while the rest of your curls are left free to frame your face. This takes just minutes to create, and it can be worn anytime, any day of the week.

TRY THIS
Go for a pop of color on the lips—depending on the season, you can go light or dark—and brush a little mascara along both top and bottom lashes for a doll-like effect.

SEE ALSO
Messy bun, pages 108–09
Double topknots, pages 124–25

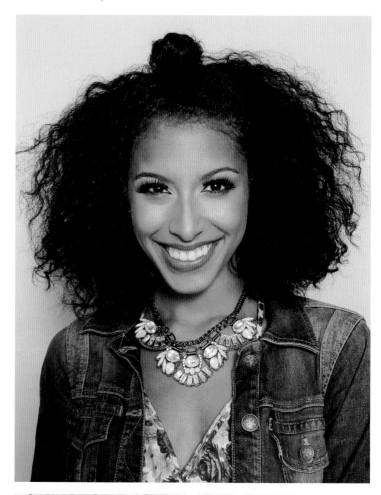

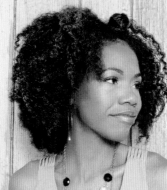

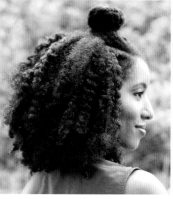

HOW TO DO IT

WHAT YOU NEED

- Comb
- Hair tie
- Bobby pins

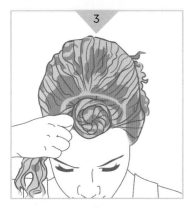
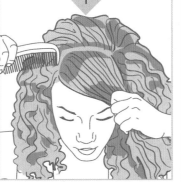
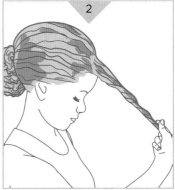
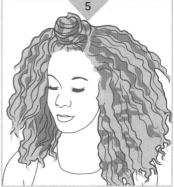
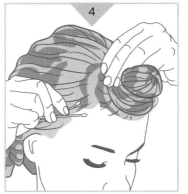

1. Using a comb, separate out a square section of hair at your forehead for your topknot. Gather the rest of your hair into a low ponytail for now to keep it out of the way.

2. Starting at the roots of the square section, begin twisting the hair until you've reached the ends.

3. Once the twist is complete, start twirling it round in a circular motion to form your bun. When it's the size and shape you want, secure it with a tie, wrapping the ends around the tie.

4. For extra security, slide bobby pins underneath the bun, distributing them evenly around the outside.

5. Finish by releasing the rest of your hair and pulling it forward over your shoulders if it's long enough.

TOP TIP

This style does not need to be perfect in any way. The bun should be small and messy, so just play around with it until you achieve the effect you want.

CURLY BEEHIVE BOUFFANT

BEST FOR
Medium to long hair

ACCESSORIES
Studded earrings and
a statement necklace.

DIFFICULTY LEVEL
Hard

ASSISTANCE NEEDED?
No

I adore this classic style. It just
screams '60s. You'll probably
need to have a few goes before
you perfect this look, but stick
with it—if you have a love for
retro hairstyles, you definitely
need to master this one. Wear
it to a cocktail party or a formal
event and you'll definitely turn
heads. It's also a great style to
have up your sleeve if you have
a costume party coming up that
calls for retro styling.

TRY THIS
Smudge some liner along your
eyes and then use a powder to
soften the look. Keep your lips
soft and pretty—opt for a pinky
neutral that suits your skin tone.

SEE ALSO
Twisted chignon, pages
100–01
Messy French twist, pages
170–71

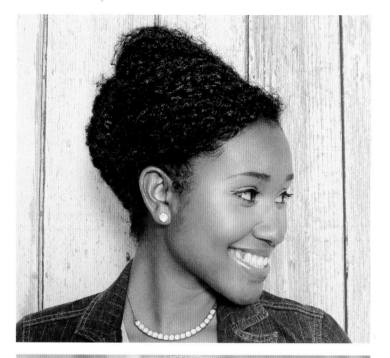

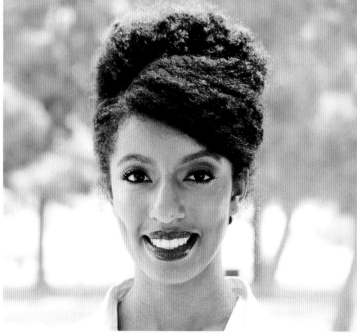

HOW TO DO IT

WHAT YOU NEED

- Bobby pins
- Hairspray (optional)

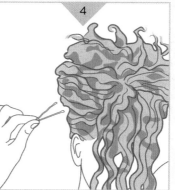

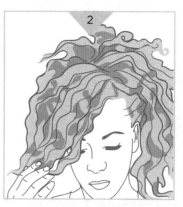

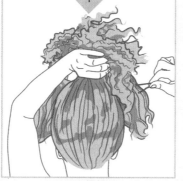

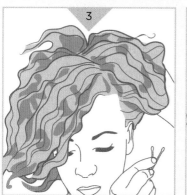

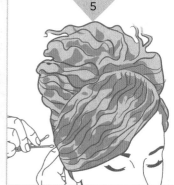

1. Gather your hair up from the back and use a good handful of bobby pins to hold it in place.

2. Your sides should now be hanging down as shown.

3. Pin one side up, folding in any stray hairs or loose ends; use as many pins as you need to keep the hair secure.

4. Now repeat the same with the other side, leaving just the hair at the very front hanging free.

5. Finally, sweep the front section of hair to one side, pinning it in place behind your ear. At this point you can also give everything a quick check, adding pins in places if you need to perfect the shape.

TOP TIP

Updos have a tendency to fall flat after a few hours' wear. Since this one relies on just pins to hold it in place, you should set it with plenty of hairspray if you plan to be out late!

DOUBLE TOPKNOTS

BEST FOR
Medium to long hair

ACCESSORIES
Since your hair is kept cleanly away from your face, add statement pieces like a necklace and/or earrings for extra impact.

DIFFICULTY LEVEL
Easy

ASSISTANCE NEEDED?
No

Double topknots are really popular right now, and are a fun choice for any curly who wants to try something new. This hairstyle is also super easy to create. The size of the topknots is entirely up to you.

TRY THIS
If the double topknots shown here are not your style, why not try a simple central topknot instead (see page 120), leaving the rest of your hair down and swept behind your shoulders?

SEE ALSO
Victory rolls, pages 116–17
Topknot, pages 120–21

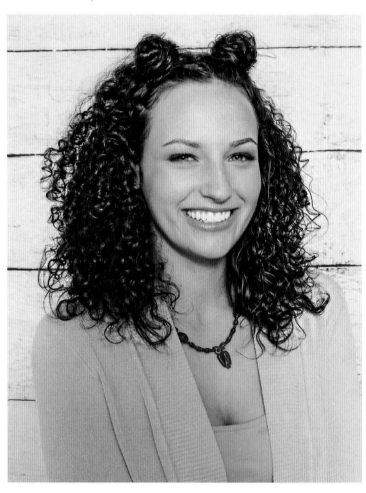

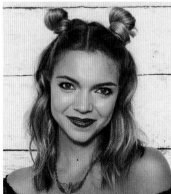

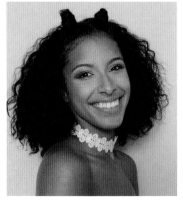

HOW TO DO IT

WHAT YOU NEED

- Curl definer
- Comb
- Hair tie
- Bobby pins
- Hairspray

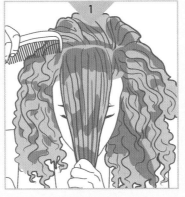

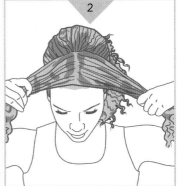

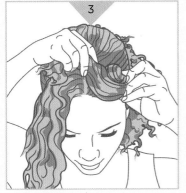

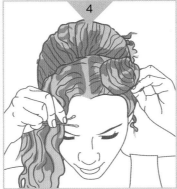

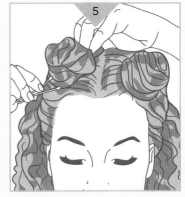

1. Apply a small amount of curl definer and use a comb to separate out a rectangular section at your forehead.

2. Divide this section into two equal halves, creating a part down the center. Gather the rest of your hair into a ponytail for now.

3. Use your fingers to roll up the first section, coiling it up into a firm topknot that sits neatly against your head. (Refer to the instructions on page 121 for extra guidance.)

4. Secure the topknot with bobby pins all the way round, sliding them underneath the topknot so that they remain hidden.

5. Now create the second topknot. Finish by gently smoothing a tiny bit of curl definer around the edges of the topknots for a more polished appearance, then set with hairspray.

TOP TIP

Make sure your topknots are as symmetrical as possible. Check the second one against the first as you work, and manipulate the shape with extra bobby pins if you need to.

HIGH BUN WITH CROWN BRAID

BEST FOR
Medium to long hair

ACCESSORIES
Go light on this one. Just add a bit of jewelry if you think you need it—a simple, thin necklace keeps the look dainty.

DIFFICULTY LEVEL
Medium

ASSISTANCE NEEDED?
No

Braids and bun just do it for me. They're the perfect pairing, and the ideal way to go when you're feeling bored with your everyday bun. A high bun lifts your hair away from your face in a flattering way, and the braids give it a flirty, fun feel. It may take a bit of practice to get the hang of this one, but it will be worth it!

TRY THIS
This style is simple and pretty, so complement it with a soft, glam look—think highlighted cheeks, a peachy cheek-and-lip combo, and a little mascara.

SEE ALSO
Curly bun with faux bangs, pages 114–15
Low bun with rolled bangs, pages 118–19

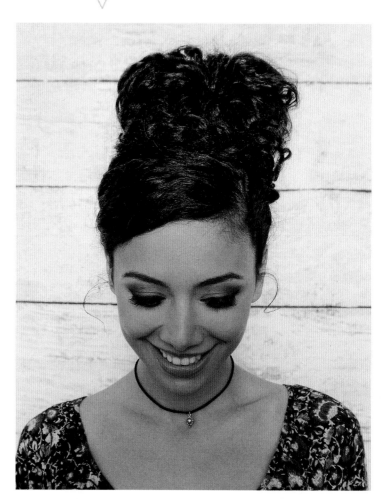

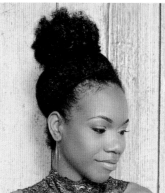

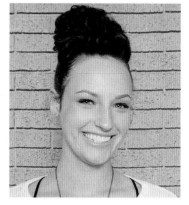

HOW TO DO IT

WHAT YOU NEED

- Hair ties
- Bobby pins

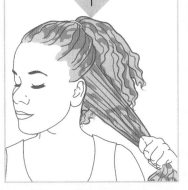

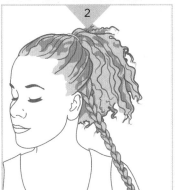

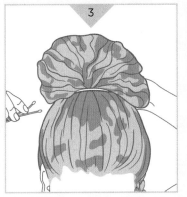

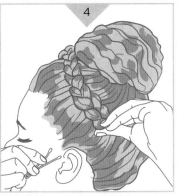

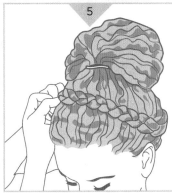

1. Separate out a medium-sized section of hair from behind one ear, then gather the rest of your hair up into a high ponytail.

2. Now take the reserved section and form a braid, securing it with a hair tie.

3. Wrap the hair of your ponytail into a bun and secure it in place with another tie. You may also need to use a bobby pin or two to perfect the shape or catch any unwanted stray hairs.

4. Take your braid and wind it up and over your head. Insert some bobby pins underneath the start of the braid so that it lays flat against your head.

5. Finish by tucking the end of the braid behind your opposite ear, securing it with a few more pins.

TOP TIP

If you'd like a thicker-looking braid, gently pull its strands apart to "fatten" it before winding it up over your head.

SIDE BUN WITH TWISTED BANGS

BEST FOR
Medium to long hair

ACCESSORIES
Glam up this 'do with a chic headband. Or add some bun jewelry or festive bobby pins to make it really pop.

DIFFICULTY LEVEL
Medium

ASSISTANCE NEEDED?
No

I love the originality of this style. It's great for girls who love a good twist and can appreciate the bun life. After a few practice runs, the flat twist becomes incredibly easy to create, and it really opens up the facial area, bringing attention to your features. This is also a great "protective" style—you can leave it in for a few days if your hair needs a bit of a break from constant styling.

TRY THIS
A bold lip and neutral eyes will really make this style pop!

▶ **SEE ALSO**
Curly bun with faux bangs, pages 114–15
High bun with crown braid, pages 126–27

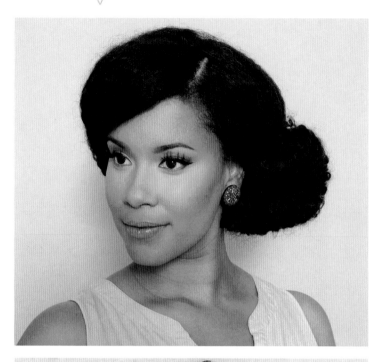

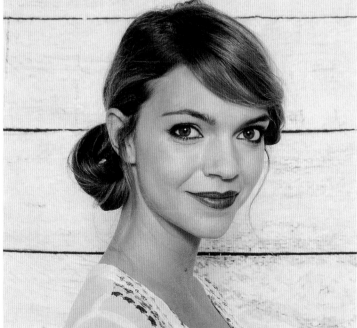

HOW TO DO IT

WHAT YOU NEED

- Comb
- Hair tie
- Bobby pins
- Hair serum

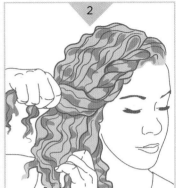

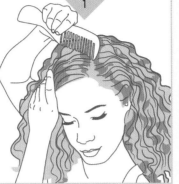

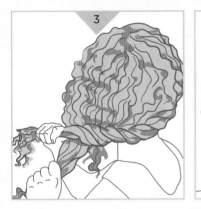

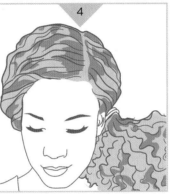

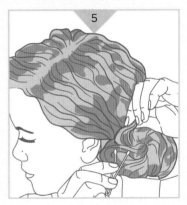

1. Create a part on your desired side with a comb, then pull the larger of the two sections forward to prepare the hair for twisting.

2. Starting at the part, begin flat-twisting your hair, following the instructions on page 50.

3. Work down and around to the far side. When you reach the back of your head you'll have to switch your hands over to the other side of your head to finish the twist.

4. Secure the twist with a hair tie.

5. Finish by wrapping your ponytail up into a bun, securing it with pins. Use some hair serum to smooth any flyaways, and catch any stray strands with extra pins if you need to.

TOP TIP

When you have completed this style, you can create a slightly more relaxed effect by gently pulling on your twist so that it flops slightly along the forehead and around the ears.

TRIPLE LOW BUNS

ACCESSORIES
As with the other low buns in this book, a headband is your best option. Choose something vivid to keep things lively!

DIFFICULTY LEVEL
Easy

ASSISTANCE NEEDED?
No

If you're looking for something fresh, these triple low buns are the perfect choice! They are casual enough to please the simple-istas among you, though their playful edge means that they are also dressy enough to sport on a special occasion. They will show off any curl type to best advantage.

TRY THIS
Since this style keeps your hair away from your face, this is the time to accentuate your features. Use a matte contour along your hairline and cheekbones, mascara for your lashes, and a bold lip color.

SEE ALSO
Halo bun, pages 96–97
Double topknots, pages 124–25

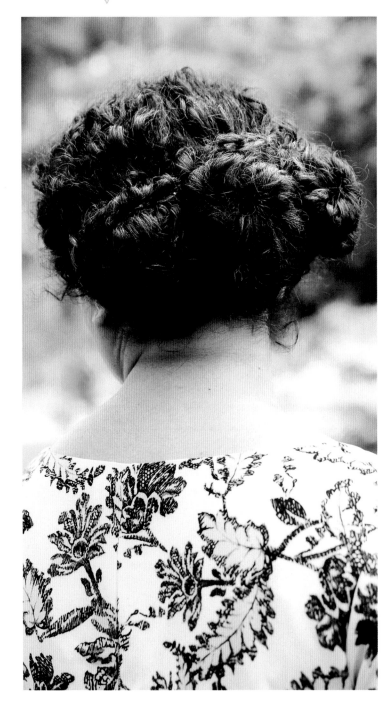

HOW TO DO IT

WHAT YOU NEED

- Hair ties
- Bobby pins
- Hairspray (optional)

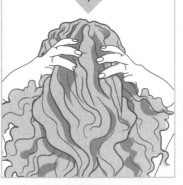

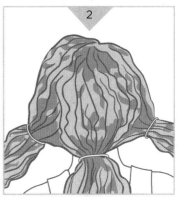

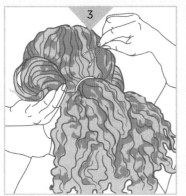

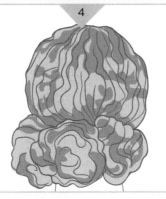

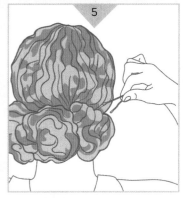

1. Gather up all of your hair and bring it back to your nape.

2. Now section off three equal parts for the buns and secure each third with a hair tie.

3. Starting on the left, wrap the hair of your ponytail around the hair tie into a loose bun and secure it in place with pins.

4. Now do the same with the other two ponytails, making sure you slide enough pins under each bun to keep them secure.

5. Use two mirrors placed opposite each other to check that all three buns are symmetrical and equally sized. Then, when you are satisfied, use a few extra pins to catch any last stray hairs, taking care not to alter the position of the buns.

TOP TIP

If the weight of the buns pulls your hair flat on top, lift the hair around the buns to free it up a bit. This will also create the illusion of thicker hair. Set the look with hairspray once you're done.

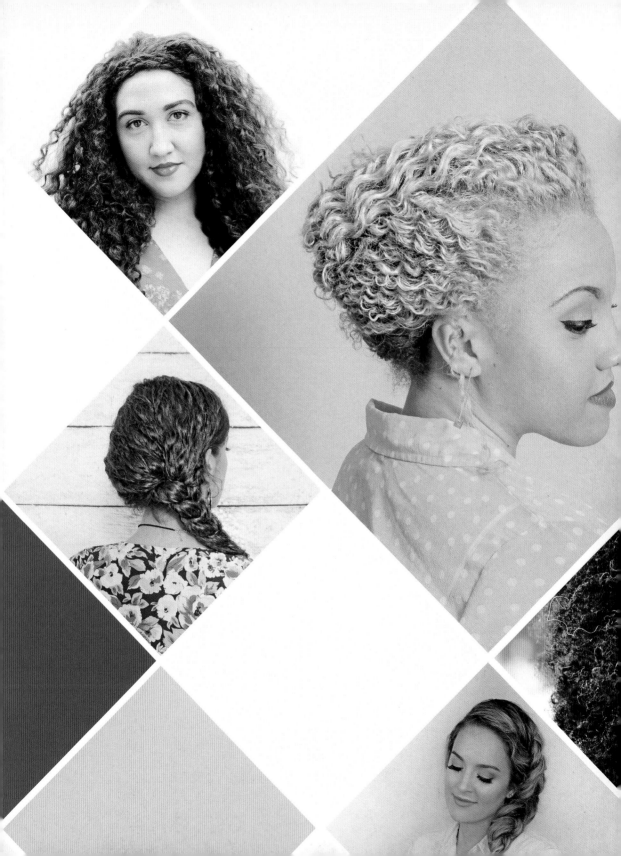

BRAIDS AND TWISTS

TWISTED STYLE

BEST FOR
Long hair

ACCESSORIES
Most of the drama of this look is at the back, so bring attention to your face with a statement necklace or earrings.

DIFFICULTY LEVEL
Medium

ASSISTANCE NEEDED?
No

How cute is this hairstyle? The twisted strands not only create a beautiful design, they also provide a handy bit of volume right round your head, whether worn with wet or dry hair. This is a style that's demure enough for everyday occasions, yet provides plenty of visual interest for those who are looking!

TRY THIS
If you want to give this a more dressy spin, slide some flowers or shimmery pins into the twists. You can also wear this style to the side—simply direct each twist toward the left or right of your head and pin it in place there, as shown on this page.

SEE ALSO
Twisted chignon, pages 100–01
Curly beehive bouffant, pages 122–23

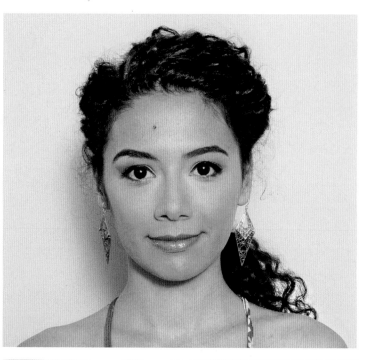

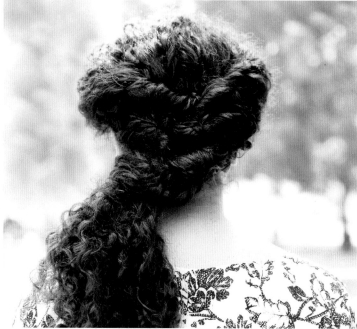

HOW TO DO IT

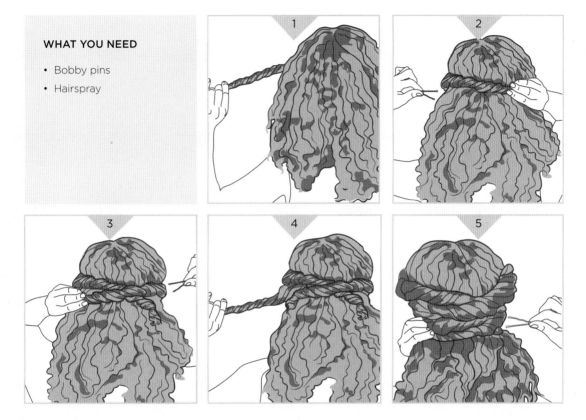

WHAT YOU NEED

- Bobby pins
- Hairspray

1. Begin by grabbing a medium-sized strand of hair from the front left side of your head. Twist the strand thoroughly, from the roots to the ends.

2. Now pass the twist across the back of your head, toward the opposite side, and secure it in place with bobby pins.

3. Repeat the same thing on the other side of your head, twisting a strand and bringing it over past the center back. Overlap the previous twist, and secure this second twist with bobby pins.

4. Now repeat Steps 2 and 3 with a fresh strand of hair from the left, taken from just below the previous strand.

5. Complete the style by repeating Steps 2 and 3 with a final strand of hair from the right. Use hairspray to keep this look in place all day.

TOP TIP

Be patient and make sure each twist feels secure before you move on to the next one. This will save you time in the long run. Use as many pins as you need to achieve this—each new twist will conveniently hide the pins of the previous one.

LOW TWISTED CURLS

BEST FOR
Medium to long hair

ACCESSORIES
If you're heading to a date or a dance, why not slide a flower behind your exposed ear to dress this look up?

DIFFICULTY LEVEL
Medium

ASSISTANCE NEEDED?
No

Stuck in a hair rut? These low twisted curls may be just what you need to get out of it! This style is much easier than it looks, too. The chunky twists give the style character and dimension, while the sideswept placement keeps it soft and feminine.

TRY THIS
Simpy changing where you create your part to begin with will give you different options for this 'do—you can try a middle part instead of the side part used here. You can even create a part on the far side and twist right across your forehead and down the other side.

SEE ALSO
Twisted style, pages 134–35
Half twists, pages 140–41

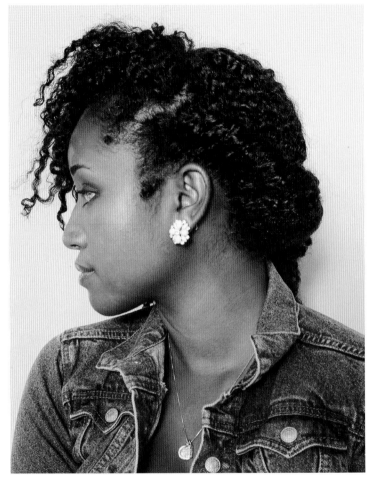

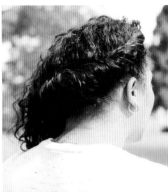

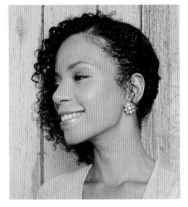

136

HOW TO DO IT

WHAT YOU NEED

- Comb
- Bobby pins
- Hairspray

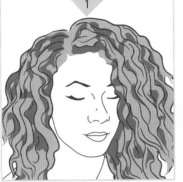

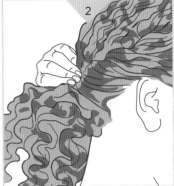

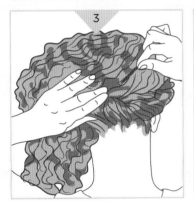

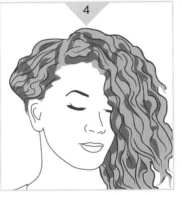

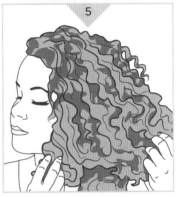

1. Use a comb to create a small side part on your right side (or left, if you prefer), running from your hairline back to your crown. If you want the finished look to have a bit of extra volume, try backcombing the roots before you begin.

2. Now take the hair on the right side of your face and begin twisting it inward and down along the side of your head, incorporating the hair along your hairline as you go.

3. Keep twisting right round until you reach the far side of your neck, then secure it here with plenty of bobby pins.

4. Now sweep your hair forward over your other shoulder.

5. Finish by running your fingers through your curls to add even more volume, and spritz on some hairspray for extra hold.

TOP TIP

While twisting, it's easy to lose the shape of your twist; you may need to start over a few times when you first try this style. To avoid too much trial and error, try pinning your hair as you go so that it's firmly held in place at every point.

TRIPLE CROWN TWISTS

BEST FOR
All hair lengths

ACCESSORIES
Since the crown twists are the focus here, choose jewelry if you want to accessorize. A pair of delicate dangly earrings can really pretty up this style.

DIFFICULTY LEVEL
Easy

ASSISTANCE NEEDED?
No

Your hair is your crown, and so you should wear it fabulously, every day! This style offers twin benefits—it keeps your hair away from your face, and makes the most of your curls by leaving the rest of your hair free. Every length and curl type will look great with this one, and it is super easy to create.

TRY THIS
Makeup for this look depends entirely on your mood. If you would like an understated look you can go completely natural, or perhaps add a lip color and a bronzer or matte contour color for your cheeks.

▷ **SEE ALSO**
Half twists, pages 140–41
Crown braids, pages 156–57

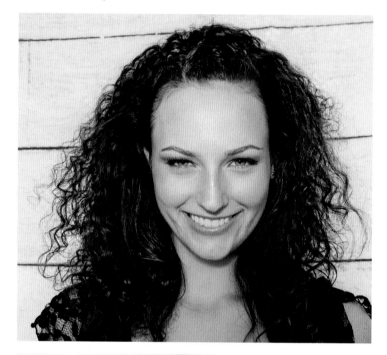

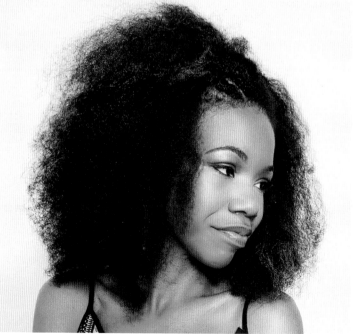

HOW TO DO IT

WHAT YOU NEED

- Hair tie
- Bobby pins
- Comb

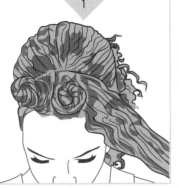

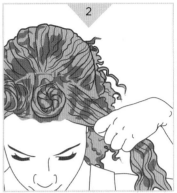

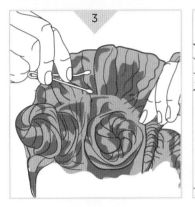

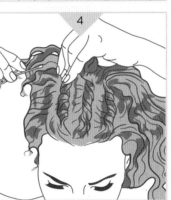

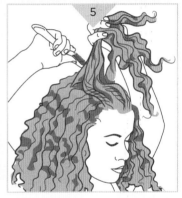

1. Use a comb to separate out a square section of hair at your forehead. Tie the rest of your hair out of the way for now, then divide the top section into three equal parts. Twist two of these up and out of the way, and leave the third hanging freely.

2. Twist this first section from the roots. The twist should begin at your hairline, then run back toward the part.

3. Once you reach the part, secure the twist with some bobby pins, letting the rest of the hair strand hang free. If your hair is quite dense, you may need to use quite a few pins.

4. Now repeat the same process with the other two sections.

5. Release the rest of your hair and tease it a bit at the roots. You want to achieve volume by focusing solely on the roots; combing all the way through the hair can cause frizziness.

TOP TIP

Twists aren't always created equal! If you're having trouble keeping the twists tight and secure, try holding the twist firmly and constantly with one hand while you pin with the other. Crisscrossing the pins will also give you the best hold.

HALF TWISTS

BEST FOR
All hair lengths

ACCESSORIES
For a night out, try inserting a few colorful pins or clips along each twist for a festive touch.

DIFFICULTY LEVEL
Easy

ASSISTANCE NEEDED?
No

Looking for a new everyday 'do? Maybe you want a style where your curls aren't flopping in your face all the time. I get it! This style is easy enough for anyone to create, and it works well regardless of hair length or curl type. It's versatile, too—you can wear this to school, for a dinner date, or even a night on the town with your BFFs.

TRY THIS
You can really go in any direction with your makeup here, but since this is a simple style, I stick to highlighting and contouring, a bit of mascara, and keeping it neutral on the lips.

SEE ALSO
Victory rolls, pages 116–17
Double side braids, pages 144–45

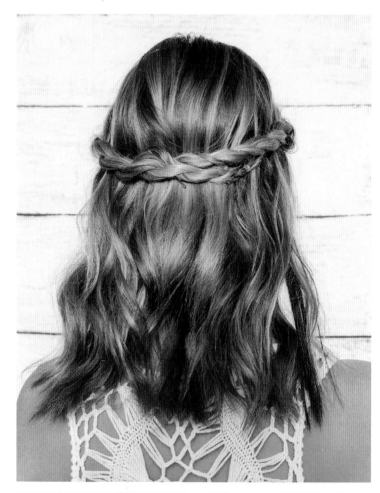

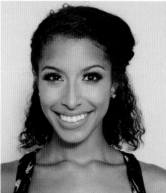

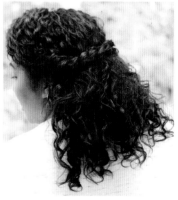

HOW TO DO IT

WHAT YOU NEED

- Comb
- Hair tie
- Bobby pins
- Curl definer (optional)

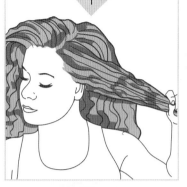

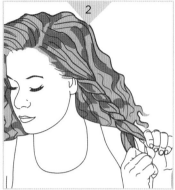

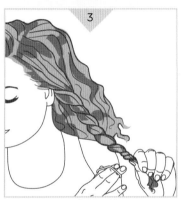

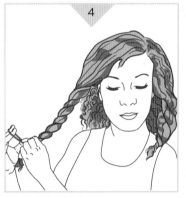

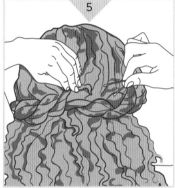

1. Use a comb to part your hair as desired, then separate out a medium-sized section from one side.

2. Divide this section into two equal strands and create a simple two-strand twist (see pages 48–49). Work all the way from the roots to the ends of the hair.

3. Secure the end of the twist with a hair tie.

4. Now grab an equal-sized section of hair on the other side of your part and repeat Steps 2 and 3.

5. Finish off by taking the ends of both twists and bringing them to the back of your head. Overlap them and then secure each one by carefully sliding bobby pins underneath them.

TOP TIP

For wider twists that use the same amount of hair, try gently lifting and pulling the twists apart once they've been pinned in place. Be careful not to dislodge the pins, though! You can also use a small amount of curl definer to help keep this style in place all day.

FRENCH BRAID

BEST FOR

Long hair

ACCESSORIES

You won't want to take too much attention away from the braid itself, so why not try something like a pair of small hoop earrings?

DIFFICULTY LEVEL

Medium/hard

ASSISTANCE NEEDED?

An extra pair of hands can help first time round.

A classic French braid should be on every girl's "must try" list. Braids of any kind are always fab and can be worn anywhere, from the beach to the office. Wear a single French braid, feed one into a ponytail, or use one in a half-up half-down style—the goal here is to be as creative as you like. The only rule is that you have fun while you're doing it!

TRY THIS

Eyeliner, bold lashes, and a pop of color on the lips will rock the socks off this style!

SEE ALSO

Jumbo Dutch braid, pages 148–49
Asymmetric braid, pages 160–61

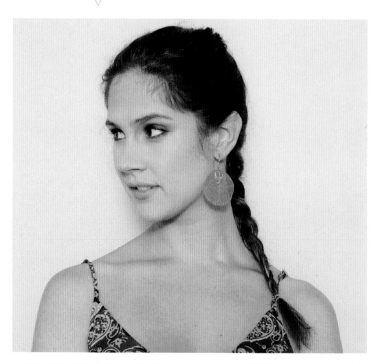

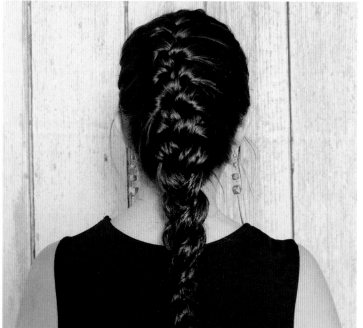

HOW TO DO IT

WHAT YOU NEED

- Hair tie
- Hairspray

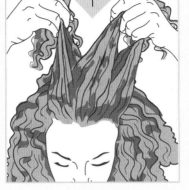

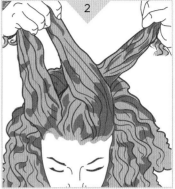

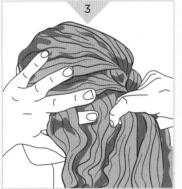

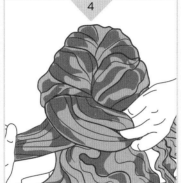

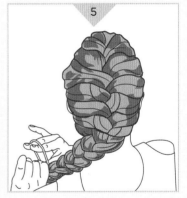

1. Separate out a section of hair at your forehead. Divide this into three equal strands, holding two strands of hair with your left hand and the third with your right.

2. Take the leftmost strand and cross it over the middle strand. The left strand will become the new middle strand. Grip this new middle strand with your right hand.

3. Repeat Step 2 with the strand on the right to complete the first segment of the braid. Continue in this way, but as you progress, feed in a fresh section of hair from the side of your head into the side strand you are working.

4. Repeat this process, incorporating hair from either side as you go, making sure your braid stays centered at the back.

5. When you reach your neck, continue with a regular braid, then secure the end with a hair tie. Finish with hairspray.

TOP TIP

Remember that slow and steady wins the race—really take the time to master this technique. You can also experiment with using your left and right hand to find the holding method that works best for you. You'll be a pro before you know it!

DOUBLE SIDE BRAIDS

BEST FOR
All hair lengths

ACCESSORIES
Jazz up your braids with some fancy bobby pins or a bit of hair jewelry. Long, dangly earrings can also be a great addition.

DIFFICULTY LEVEL
Medium/hard

ASSISTANCE NEEDED?
No

Double side braids are so simple and cute. They have an everyday vibe but can also be worn on more festive occasions, and the two braids create a headband effect that keeps your curls conveniently away from your face. Any length of hair and any curl type can wear this look, but if you have shorter hair, you may want to lift your curls at the roots for more volume.

TRY THIS
You won't want to interfere with the playful simplicity of this hairstyle. Keep any makeup neutral, soft, and pretty.

SEE ALSO
Half twists, pages 140–41
Crown braids, pages 156–57

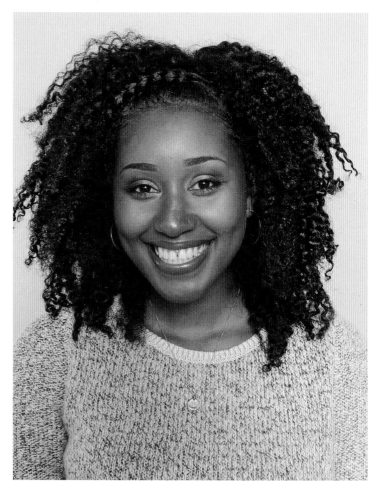

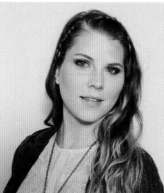

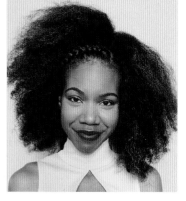

HOW TO DO IT

WHAT YOU NEED

- Curl definer
- Hair ties

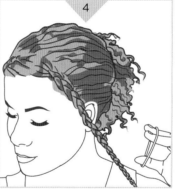

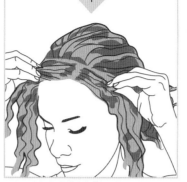

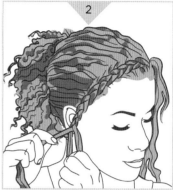

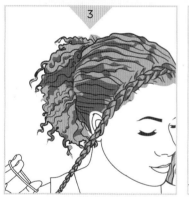

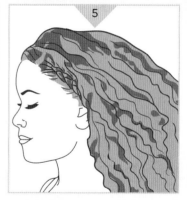

1. To show off your curls at their best use a curl definer before starting this style. Separate out a thin section of hair along your hairline, running from the front of one ear across to the other. Tie the rest of your hair out of the way, then divide the top section in two, slightly to the side of center.

2. Begin cornrowing one section from the part down to the ear—this involves forming a Dutch braid (see page 149) that sits close to the scalp.

3. Once you reach the ear, continue the braid to the ends and then secure it with a hair tie.

4. Repeat the same process on the second section of hair.

5. Now release the rest of your hair. Tuck the ends of the two braids behind your ears, out of sight, then fluff up your curls and pull them forward over your ears.

TOP TIP

If your hair curls up tightly, try stretching it a bit by using the two-strand twist-out method the night before you want to wear this style (see pages 48–49 for instructions).

FISHTAIL BRAID

BEST FOR
Long hair

ACCESSORIES
Since this hairstyle is dramatic enough on its own, you'll need nothing more than some simple jewelry. A long, thin necklace can work well. If you want to dress it up, give it a boho feel with a chunky bracelet.

DIFFICULTY LEVEL
Medium

ASSISTANCE NEEDED?
No

While I love braids of all shapes and forms, a fishtail is what I choose when I want something chic, but with a bit more edge. Curls are a bonus because they give this style a messiness that really works! Although this is a complex-looking braid, it's actually a whole lot easier than it looks. If you know how to braid, you'll pick it up in no time.

TRY THIS
Enhance your features with highlighting and contouring, followed by a soft blush-and-lip combo, and some mascara on both top and bottom lashes.

SEE ALSO
Side braid, pages 154–55
Boho fishtail, pages 158–59

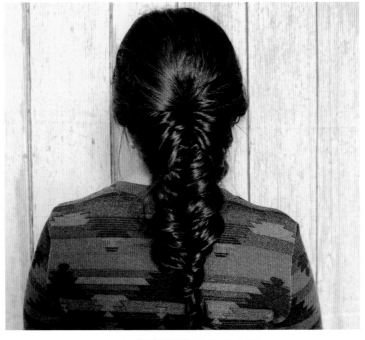

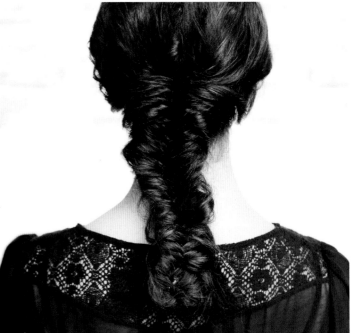

HOW TO DO IT

WHAT YOU NEED

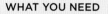

- Comb
- Hair tie

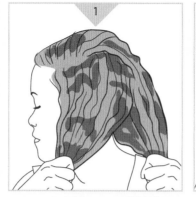

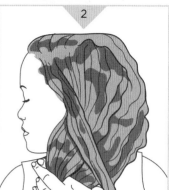

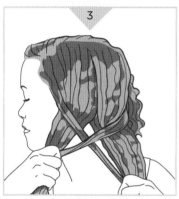

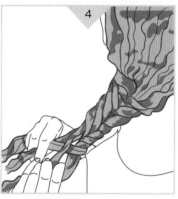

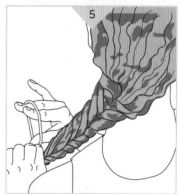

1. Use a comb to gather all of your hair into a low ponytail at the back of your head. Divide the hair into two equal sections.

2. Take a small strand of hair from the outer edge of the one section of hair and cross it over to join the other section.

3. Now repeat Step 2, this time taking a small strand of hair from the outside edge of the second section, and crossing it over to join the first section. You will now see the beginnings of your fishtail pattern.

4. Continue with this method, crossing strands from the outside edge of each section in turn until you reach the ends.

5. Secure the completed fishtail braid with a hair tie.

TOP TIP

Once your braid is complete, you can make the fishtail pattern more prominent by pulling the strands apart slightly. Start at the base of the ponytail and work your way down to the ends.

JUMBO DUTCH BRAID

BEST FOR

Long hair

ACCESSORIES

As with the fishtail braid, you won't want to detract from the braid itself, so if you want extra pizzazz, add earrings—studs for everyday, or large hoops for street-style vibes.

DIFFICULTY LEVEL

Medium/hard

ASSISTANCE NEEDED?

An extra pair of hands can help first time round.

If your hair is a bit overworked, a jumbo Dutch braid offers the perfect solution. Since this style lasts for a few days, you can stop thinking about your hair and give it a well-earned rest, too! After a couple of goes you'll be able to create it in no time, and you'll find it's versatile enough to take you from office to gym, and back again.

TRY THIS

A Dutch braid gives you a little more definition and bulk than a French braid, so a bold eye-and-lip combo can be the perfect complement.

SEE ALSO

French braid, pages 142–43
Fishtail braid, pages 146–47

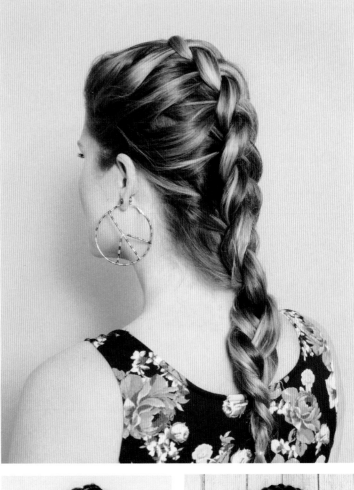

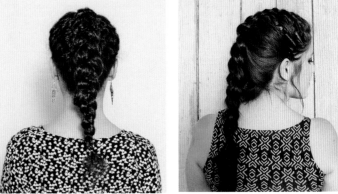

HOW TO DO IT

WHAT YOU NEED

- Hair tie
- Hairspray (optional)

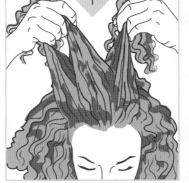

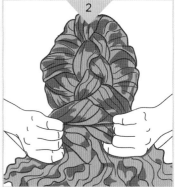

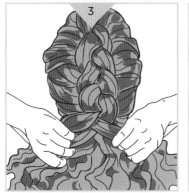

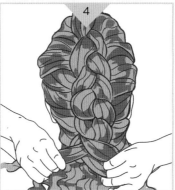

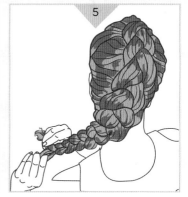

1. Grab three strands of hair at the top of your head, holding two strands with your right hand, and the third with your left.

2. Unlike a French braid, which is inverted, a Dutch braid sits on top of your hair. Take the strand on your right and cross it under the middle strand to become the new middle strand. Grip it with your other hand. Repeat the same with the left strand to complete the first segment of the braid. Continue in this way, but as you progress, feed in fresh sections of hair from the side of your head into each side strand as you go.

3. Continue down, keeping the braid in a central position.

4. Incorporate the last bits of free hair at the nape.

5. Keep braiding to the ends, then secure it with a tie. If your hair falls out of braids easily you can set this style with hairspray.

TOP TIP

Don't put yourself under pressure to create this style at a moment's notice. Instead, try practicing both this and the French braiding technique (page 143) in your downtime.

HALF FRENCH TWIST

BEST FOR
All hair lengths

ACCESSORIES
Try some ear cuffs if you fancy wearing a bit of jewelry. Alternatively, slip a bold hair pin or slide into your twist.

DIFFICULTY LEVEL
Easy

ASSISTANCE NEEDED?
No

This is a fresh take on the standard French twist (see page 170), a half-up half-down variation that manages to be both flirty and sophisticated. With this version you get the classic look of a French twist, but with a lot less work—simply twist and pin and you've got this style down!

TRY THIS
During the day, opt for natural makeup. Think eyeliner, mascara, and your favorite lip color. For special occasions, introduce a smoky eye to keep the focus on your face.

SEE ALSO
Twisted half-up ponytail, pages 78–79
Messy French twist, pages 170–71

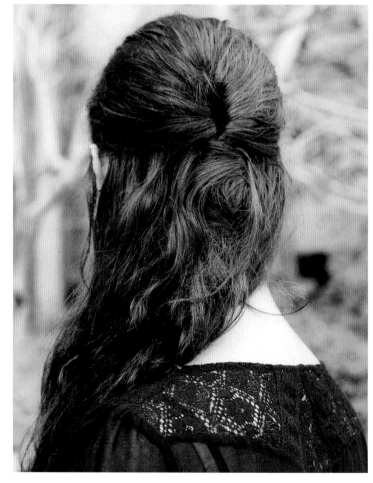

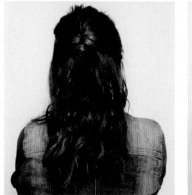

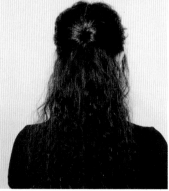

HOW TO DO IT

WHAT YOU NEED

- Comb
- Hair tie
- Bobby pins
- Hairspray

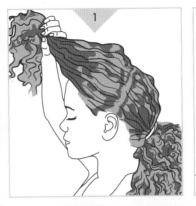

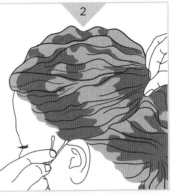

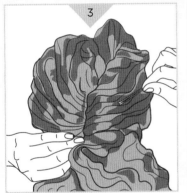

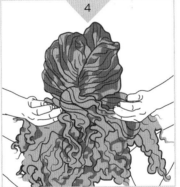

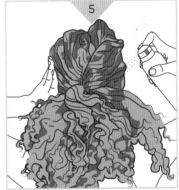

1. Use a comb to part your hair horizontally straight across the crown. Tie the lower section out of the way with a hair tie while you work on the top half.

2. Divide the top section in half. Take the half on your left, sweep it to the center back of your head, then secure it with pins.

3. Now twist the right half across the back center, twisting it underneath and securing it with pins all the way down the join. The twist should completely cover the pins used in Step 2.

4. Release the bottom section of hair and fluff up your curls, working gently so as to avoid dislodging any pins.

5. Finally, set your 'do with hairspray to give it some extra hold throughout the day. Use your fingers to tweak and perfect the style as you spray.

TOP TIP

If you find it tricky to form your twist at first, try working with two mirrors placed opposite each other so that you can monitor what is happening at the back of your head. You'll soon be able to do this with your eyes closed!

CENTER BRAID

BEST FOR
All hair lengths

ACCESSORIES
You'll want your braid to be the central focus, so stick to jewelry rather than hair accessories. A strong necklace can be really effective.

DIFFICULTY LEVEL
Medium

ASSISTANCE NEEDED?
An extra pair of hands can help the first time round.

The useful thing about the center braid is that it works well on any hair texture or length. It's a particularly good choice if you have fine hair and want to add a bit more dimension to your curls. To get the most out of this style, start with second- or third-day hair, which will have more volume.

TRY THIS
Since your hair is kept away from your face, use a matte contour powder or bronzer to accentuate your facial structure.

▶ **SEE ALSO**
Crown braids, pages 156–57
Asymmetric braid, pages 160–61

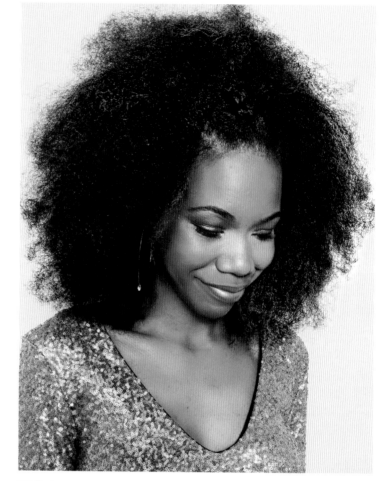

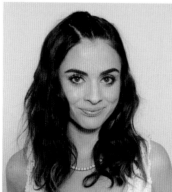

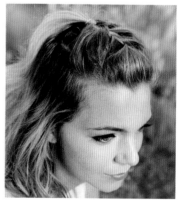

HOW TO DO IT

WHAT YOU NEED

- Comb
- Bobby pins
- Hair tie
- Hairspray

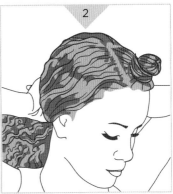
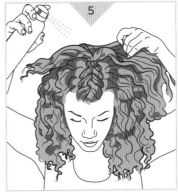
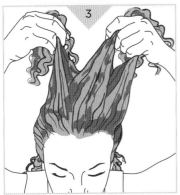
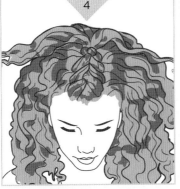
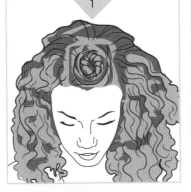

1. Use a comb to separate out a rectangular section at your forehead for your braid. Twist it up out of the way.

2. Gather the rest of your hair in a low ponytail to keep it out of the way while you work on your braid.

3. Now release your top section, divide it into three equal strands, and begin creating a French braid, following the instructions on page 143.

4. When you reach the part at the back of the top section, stop braiding and use a few bobby pins to hold the braid in place. Release the rest of your hair.

5. Use your comb or your fingers to lift a few curls at the roots to create some extra volume. A few spritzes of hairspray while doing this will keep the look intact throughout the day.

TOP TIP

For this, and other relevant styles, try substituting bobby pins for hair ties whenever you can. They are much easier to remove, so you'll spend less time pulling and tugging on your delicate curls.

SIDE BRAID

BEST FOR
Long hair

ACCESSORIES
Although some braids are best left to display themselves without accessories, this one looks great with a cute, patterned headband. Both thick and thin headbands showcase this style very well.

DIFFICULTY LEVEL
Easy

ASSISTANCE NEEDED?
No

Side braids are a handy option if you want to give your hair a break from styling for a while. Over-manipulating your curls can stunt growth and promote breakage, so it's a good idea to set them in a quick and simple style like this every now and then and then leave them be.

TRY THIS
This hairstyle is soft and pretty, so play it up by wearing your favorite lip gloss, with contour for your cheeks and mascara to make your eyes pop.

SEE ALSO
Fishtail braid, pages 146–47
Boho fishtail, pages 158–59

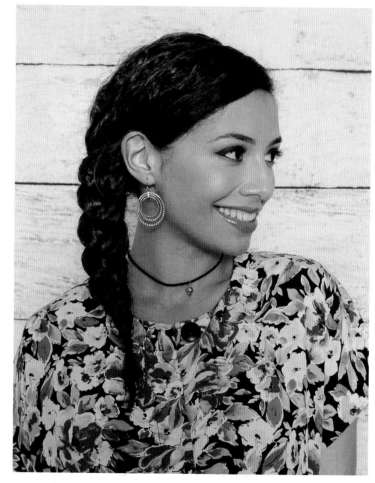

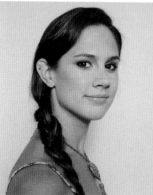

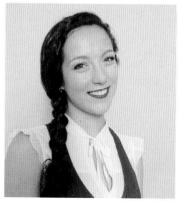

HOW TO DO IT

WHAT YOU NEED

- Comb
- Hair tie
- Bobby pins
- Hairspray

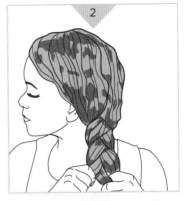

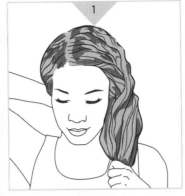

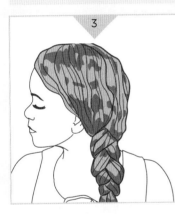

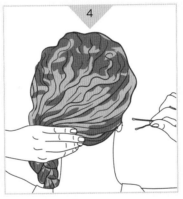

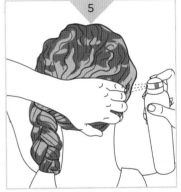

1. Gather all of your hair round to one side. Use a comb if necessary to smooth any flyaway hairs along the hairline.

2. Divide your hair into three equal sections and begin forming a simple braid.

3. Continue right to the ends, and then secure the braid with a hair tie.

4. If you are heading out you may want to grab any loose hairs around your neck and pin them in place to keep everything looking neat.

5. Finally, spray the finished look with hairspray. This will hold it in place and keep your curls from frizzing.

TOP TIP

Braids are a great protective style, so make the most of them by wearing them for a few days if you can. Your hair will thank you for the rest! Remember to wrap your hair in a silk or satin bonnet overnight, to avoid frizz and to prolong the style.

CROWN BRAIDS

BEST FOR
All hair lengths

ACCESSORIES
Once again, the braids provide the visual interest with this style, so limit yourself to some jewelry to set it off—a simple necklace or earrings would be best.

DIFFICULTY LEVEL
Easy

ASSISTANCE NEEDED?
No

Unleash your inner goddess with this hairstyle! Crown braids are perfect for showing off curls, so they provide a great add-on for lots of different curly hairstyles.

TRY THIS
If you're a braid lover, add in two extra crown braids for a bolder effect. You can also gather the rest of your hair into a high or low pony for another variation.

▶ **SEE ALSO**
High bun with crown braid, pages 126–27
Triple crown twists, pages 138–39

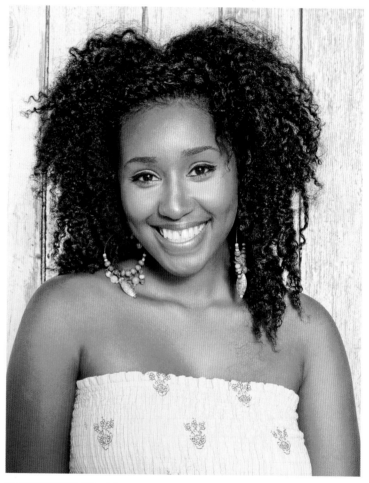

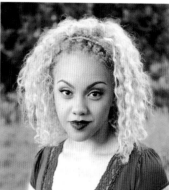

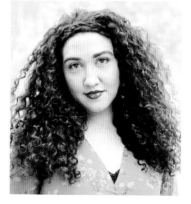

HOW TO DO IT

WHAT YOU NEED

- Hair ties
- Bobby pins
- Comb or pick
- Root booster spray (optional)

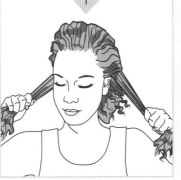

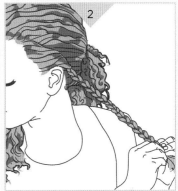

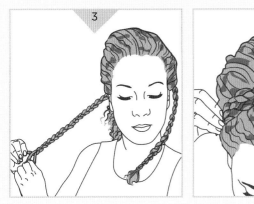

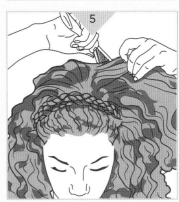

1. Grab a small section of hair from behind each of your ears and then tie the rest of your hair out of the way for now. These two sections will serve as your braids. They can be small, medium, or large, depending on how thick you want your braids to be.

2. Braid the first section until you reach the end of the hair and secure it with a hair tie.

3. Repeat this with the opposite section.

4. Now take both braids and pass them over the top of your head, running parallel to your hairline. Tuck the ends of each braid behind your ears and secure them here with bobby pins.

5. Finish off by releasing the rest of your hair, and spreading it out and forward to cover the bobby pins. Use a comb or pick to lift at the roots for more volume.

TOP TIP

Spray some root booster spray at the roots to add volume to your curls. The crown braids will naturally pull your curls forward, but a little extra volume never hurts!

BOHO FISHTAIL

BEST FOR
Long hair

ACCESSORIES
Large feather earrings or hoops would really add some street glam to this look.

DIFFICULTY LEVEL
Medium

ASSISTANCE NEEDED?
No

The messier version of the fishtail (pages 146–47), I like to think of the boho as the rebel of the braid gang. This hairstyle is very dramatic and can give the illusion of thicker, fuller hair. It's best suited to longer hair, but those of you with shorter hair needn't feel left out—adding clip-in extensions before you start will give you great results.

TRY THIS
Feeling bohemian? Add in some colorful clip-on extensions or some hair strings to give this messy look a bit of extra oomph. You can be as subtle or as bold as you like!

 SEE ALSO
Fishtail braid, pages 146–47
Sideswept braid, pages 164–65

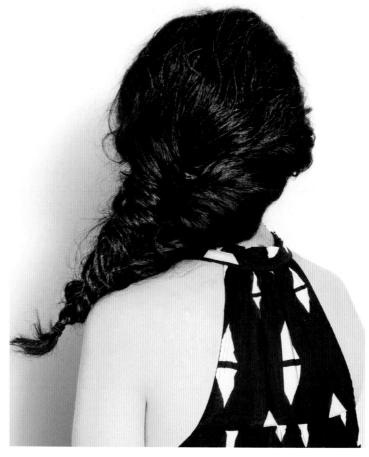

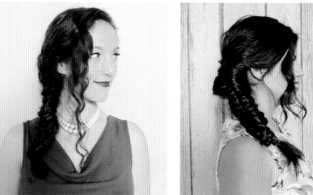

HOW TO DO IT

WHAT YOU NEED

- Comb
- Hair tie

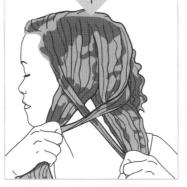

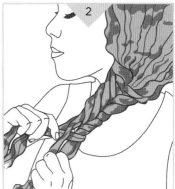

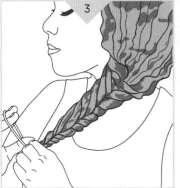

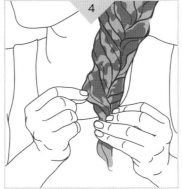

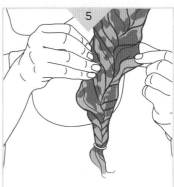

1. Gather all of your hair to the lower right (or left) side of your head using a comb. Divide the hair in half and begin the fishtail braid process, following the instructions on page 147.

2. Continue with the fishtail pattern until you reach the ends of your hair. If necessary, stop every now and then to check that both sides are even. You'll find that it also helps to work slowly.

3. Secure the end of the braid with a hair tie.

4. Holding onto the end of the braid, use your fingers to lift random strands from the braid, one at a time, to create a messy effect.

5. When you have reached the top of the braid, stop and analyze your work. Use both hands to pull out a few sections on both sides to create the thickness you need.

TOP TIP

Although you won't want to undo your braid work altogether, the more strands you tug at, the better this style will look—it's meant to be super messy!

ASYMMETRIC BRAID

BEST FOR
Long hair

ACCESSORIES
Complement the curve of this braid with some long, sleek earrings or a pair of studs.

DIFFICULTY LEVEL
Medium/hard

ASSISTANCE NEEDED?
No

I love this braided style! You can rock it Dutch style, as in the tutorial provided opposite, or French style, as shown on this page—either way it will look fabulous. I've shown you how to create a single braid that wraps right round one side of your head and draws in all of your hair, but you can also opt for a half-up half-down variation, wearing half of your hair in an asymmetric braid and keeping the lower half hanging free.

TRY THIS
Mascara and a few false lashes are a great way to emphasize your features.

▶ **SEE ALSO**
French braid, pages 142–43
Sideswept braid, pages 164–65

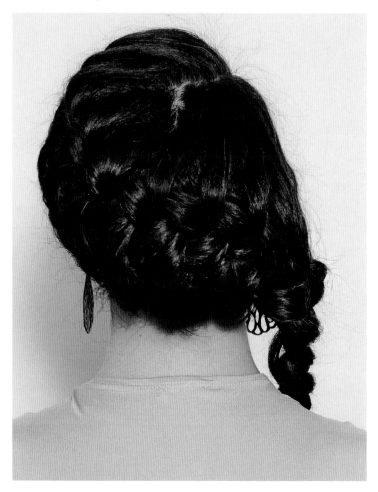

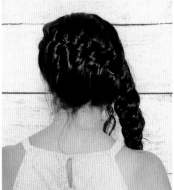

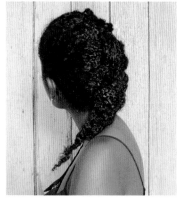

HOW TO DO IT

WHAT YOU NEED

- Curl definer
- Hair tie

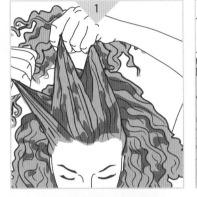
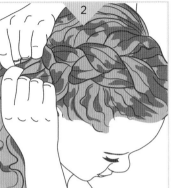
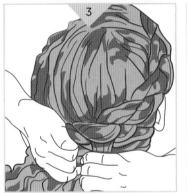
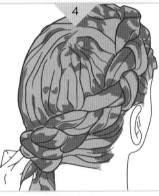
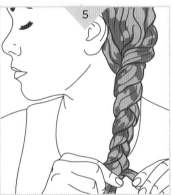

1. Run curl definer through your hair to keep it smooth. For this braid, you'll be working a Dutch braid down through your hair, working at an angle. Start by grabbing three equal-sized strands of hair at your hairline, slightly to one side.

2. Begin to form the braid following the instructions on page 149. As you progress, make sure that the braid is leaning to one side of your head. Work slowly, stopping every now and then to check that you are on track.

3. When you reach your ear, adjust your angle so that you start braiding down and round to the back of your head.

4. Once you reach your nape, begin to travel toward the other side of your head, incorporating any last bits of hair. Swap your hands to the other side of your head to complete this part.

5. Continue braiding to the ends, then secure them with a hair tie.

TOP TIP

If you want to create a slightly more boho-chic look, gently pull out some strands along the braid once it's complete. Be careful not to unravel your work, though!

CINNAMON ROLL BRAID

BEST FOR
Long hair

ACCESSORIES
A bold, blingy headband would be perfect with this style.

DIFFICULTY LEVEL
Easy

ASSISTANCE NEEDED?
No

The cinnamon roll braid is a great style to have in your collection. It can be worn as an everyday look, or created for occasions when an updo is required. It's also easy enough for girls who like a cute style but don't like the complexity of updos. If you have fine hair you'll love the way this provides a bit of extra oomph.

TRY THIS
You can opt for a smoky eye with this look, or you can keep it neutral with mascara and eyeliner only.

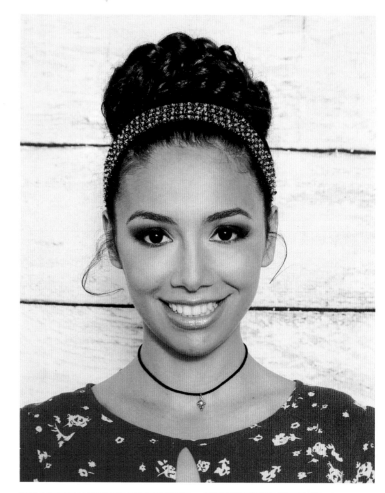

SEE ALSO
Halo bun, pages 96–97
Rope-braid bun, pages
104–05

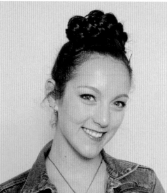
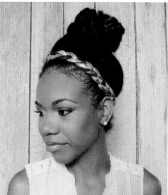

HOW TO DO IT

WHAT YOU NEED

- Hair tie
- Bobby pins
- Curl definer
- Rat-tail comb

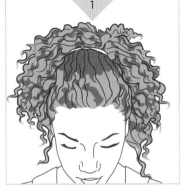

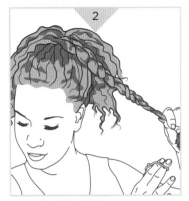

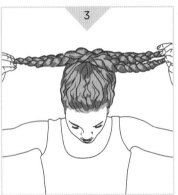

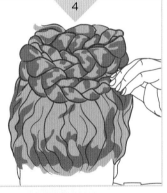

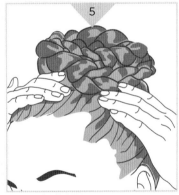

1. Start by putting your hair up into a high ponytail.

2. Divide your ponytail into three subsections. Divide one of these into three strands, then create a braid. Secure it with a hair tie.

3. Now braid the other two sections.

4. Lift the braid on your left, wrap it around the hair tie, and secure it with pins. Follow with the middle braid, wrapping it around the first braid and securing it with more pins. Finish by wrapping the final braid in the opposite direction, around the middle braid. Each braid should overlap the other to create the "cinnamon roll" effect.

5. Use a dime-sized amount of curl definer to smooth the edges of your hair. If you have trouble getting your ends to lie down, use a rat-tail comb to tuck them in place.

TOP TIP

To create a bigger bun, widen each braid with your fingers before you coil it up into the bun. Your hair will look fuller and the style will be made even more dramatic.

SIDESWEPT BRAID

BEST FOR

Medium to long hair

ACCESSORIES

Let the braid do the work with this style. All you need to add, if anything, is a simple necklace or some dangly earrings.

DIFFICULTY LEVEL

Medium

ASSISTANCE NEEDED?

No

The sideswept braid is very much like the asymmetric braid seen earlier (page 160), but this is generally done French-style. However, if you prefer the look of a Dutch-style braid, have at it—the choice is yours! This style can be worn for any occasion and looks great on all curl types.

TRY THIS

This is such a stylish hairdo that you won't want to complicate things. Try highlighting and contouring the face, but keep any makeup neutral.

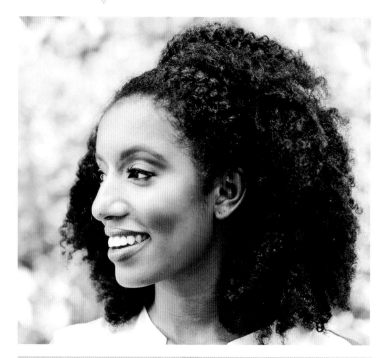

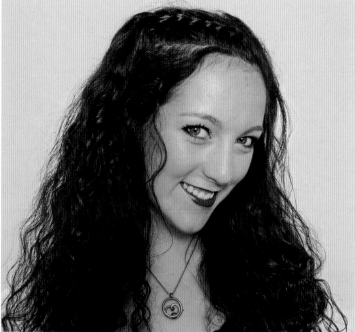

 SEE ALSO

Center braid, pages 152–53
Asymmetric braid, pages 160–61

HOW TO DO IT

WHAT YOU NEED

- Leave-in conditioner
- Bobby pins
- Wide-toothed comb
- Rat-tail comb (optional)

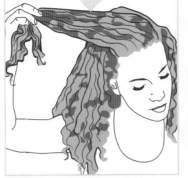

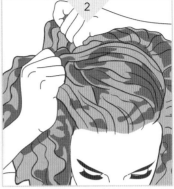

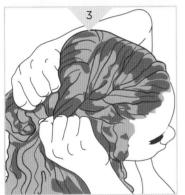

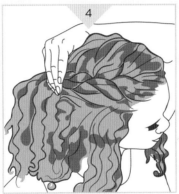

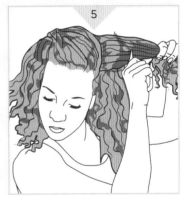

1. Smooth your hair to one side. Grab a medium-sized section for the beginning of your braid from near the top of your head. If you're starting with second- or third-day hair, spritz on a little leave-in conditioner and use your fingers to detangle this section in order to make the braiding process easier.

2. Separate the section into three equal parts and begin braiding your hair at an angle, creating a French braid (see page 143).

3. Keep braiding in this direction until you reach the crown of your head, then stop.

4. Slide some bobby pins underneath the braid to hold it in place.

5. Now use a wide-toothed comb to lift the roots of your hair everywhere else to create a bit of volume. Pull your curls forward with both hands to finish.

TOP TIP

If you want this to look more polished, use a rat-tail comb to very gently smooth out any uneven parts along the sides of your braid.

DOUBLE DUTCH BRAIDS

BEST FOR
Medium to long hair

ACCESSORIES
A statement necklace would pair well with this hairstyle.

DIFFICULTY LEVEL
Medium/hard

ASSISTANCE NEEDED?
Yes

If one Dutch braid isn't enough, try two! The more the merrier, right? Braids are always great for making the most of your curls, and doubling them up creates a stylish braided-crown effect. If you have ever had an urge to try cornrowing (forming small Dutch braids that sit close to your head), this is just the style to get started. However, if you find it hard to begin with, recruit a friend to help!

TRY THIS
Try neutral eye makeup and lips for this style.

▶ **SEE ALSO**
Jumbo Dutch braid, pages 148–49
Asymmetric braid, pages 160–61

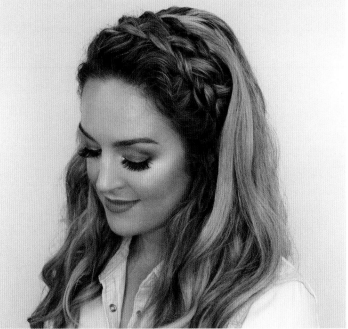

HOW TO DO IT

WHAT YOU NEED

- Comb
- Hair ties
- Bobby pins
- Curl definer (optional)

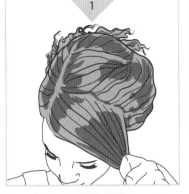

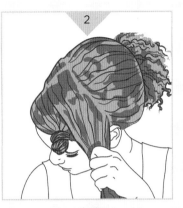

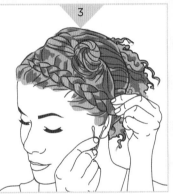

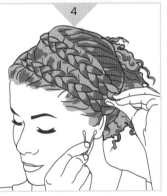

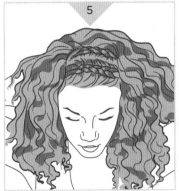

1. Create a side part using a comb, then carve out a rectangular section, running from the part to the front of your ear. Tie the rest of your hair out of the way.

2. Coil this top section up with a hair tie, then separate out a second rectangular section, starting at the side part and directly behind the first section. Secure this section with a hair tie. These two sections will be your Dutch braids.

3. Release the first section and braid down toward your ear, following the instructions for a Dutch braid on page 149. Once you reach your ear, use pins to hold it in place.

4. Now braid the second rectangular section, keeping parallel with the previous braid, and pin this in place, too.

5. Finally, release the rest of your hair and pull your curls forward so that they cover any visible bobby pins or parts.

TOP TIPS

Once finished, use your fingers to gently widen the braids for a thicker, more dramatic "headband." (Don't braid too tightly or this will be hard to do.)

If you have coarser hair, apply some curl definer along the hairline prior to braiding to keep any stubborn edge hairs in place.

DUTCH PIGTAILS

BEST FOR
Medium to long hair

ACCESSORIES
Hoop earrings will give this 'do an edgy vibe. Stud earrings can look great as well.

DIFFICULTY LEVEL
Medium/hard

ASSISTANCE NEEDED?
Yes

This hairstyle has made a comeback and the timing couldn't be more perfect. Any age and hair type can sport these braids. And if you don't have long hair, you can still make this style work for you by using hair extensions. Wear these braids to the gym, to the movies, or anywhere your heart desires!

TRY THIS
This style is so playful, I would wear only mascara and your favorite lip color to complement it. For dressier occasions, some false lashes will add drama.

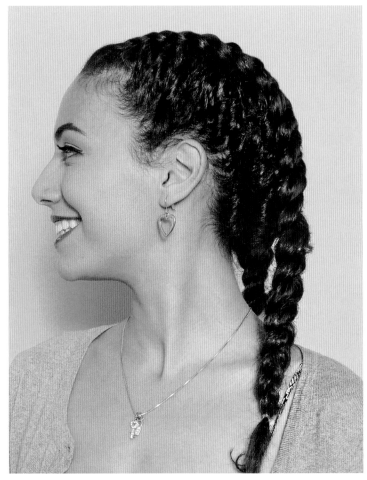

SEE ALSO
French braid, pages 142–43
Jumbo Dutch braid, pages 148–49

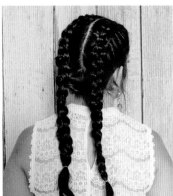

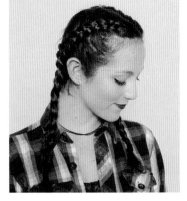

HOW TO DO IT

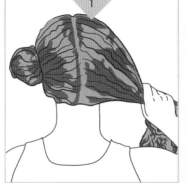

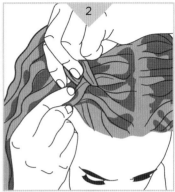

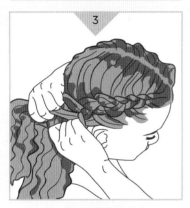

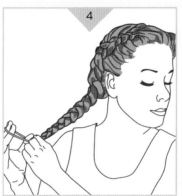

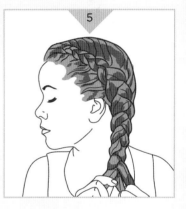

1. Use a comb to part your hair vertically into two equal halves. Secure one half off to the side with a hair tie, while you work on the other half.

2. Starting at the hairline, grab three equal-sized strands of hair and begin forming a Dutch braid down the side (see page 149 for instructions).

3. Keep braiding down toward the nape of your neck.

4. Once you reach your neck and you have incorporated all the hair on this side into the braid, continue braiding down to the ends, then secure them firmly with a hair tie.

5. Remove the hair tie from your other half and repeat Steps 2 to 4 to complete a companion pigtail.

TOP TIP

Use a rat-tail comb to gently smooth the hair along the sides of the braids in order to conceal any visible part lines.

MESSY FRENCH TWIST

BEST FOR
Medium to long hair

ACCESSORIES
Dangly or stud earrings will
work, depending on how
flamboyant you want to look.
Try a bold neck piece if you're
off to a meeting or an interview.

DIFFICULTY LEVEL
Medium

ASSISTANCE NEEDED?
No

This classic hairstyle has been
around forever, but it hasn't
aged a bit. It is such an elegant,
adaptable style, too—you can
wear it when you're hitting the
town with your girlfriends or for
a formal occasion that calls for
a fancy updo. Curls enhance the
messy, playful look of this style,
and it's very easy to create—
perfect for those who don't
like to fuss with their hair.

TRY THIS
For everyday, neutral makeup
and a pop of color on the lips
works. For special occasions,
smoky eyes and a contoured
face will take it up a notch.

▶ **SEE ALSO**
Half French twist, pages
150–51
Mini side twists, pages
174–75

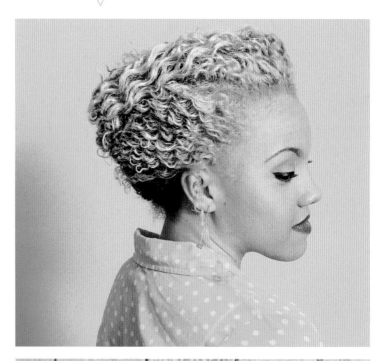

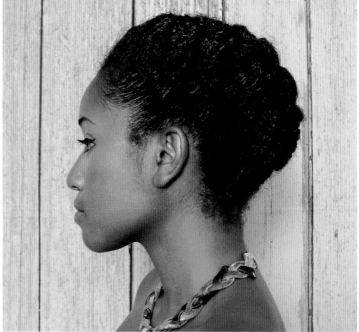

HOW TO DO IT

WHAT YOU NEED

- Curl definer
- Bobby pins
- Hairspray (optional)

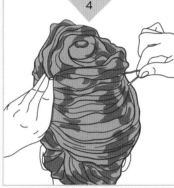

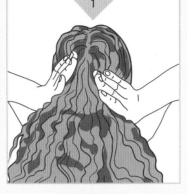

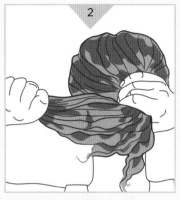

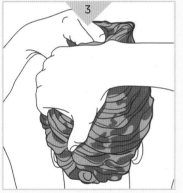

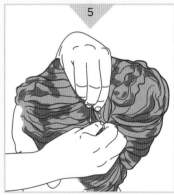

1. If you have any unruly stray hairs, smooth a bit of curl definer along the sides to hold them in place before you begin, then gather all of your hair at the back of your head.

2. Grab hold of your hair with your right hand, as if you're going to create a ponytail. While holding it here, use your left hand to lift the ends of the hair and then roll them under.

3. As you roll the ends with your left hand, use your right hand to lift and hold the shape of the twist. Play with Steps 2 and 3 for a minute to get the technique down.

4. Once the shape looks right, use one hand to slide bobby pins underneath it while you hold it in place with your other hand.

5. When the twist feels secure, you can let go and continue pinning down the join of the twist with both hands.

TOP TIP

If you have a finer curl type, you may find that you need to set this with hairspray for a more efficient hold, since it relies on just bobby pins to keep it in place.

HIGH-CROWN BRAID

BEST FOR
Long hair

ACCESSORIES
Keep it simple—a pair of stud
earrings will look great.

DIFFICULTY LEVEL
Medium/hard

ASSISTANCE NEEDED?
No

Give your French braid a run
for its money. This high-crown
variation is still perfect for
everyday wear, but it has a fun
edge, and it cleverly creates the
illusion of fuller hair with very
little effort. Forming a bun on
top of your head before you
start gives you instant height,
plus gives your hair a break from
backcombing.

TRY THIS
Don't overwhelm this everyday
style with heavy makeup. Simply
highlight your cheekbones with
a bronzer-and-blush combo,
and top it off with a soft, pretty
matte shade on your lips.

SEE ALSO
High-crown ponytail, pages
62–63
Wrapped ponytail, pages
64–65

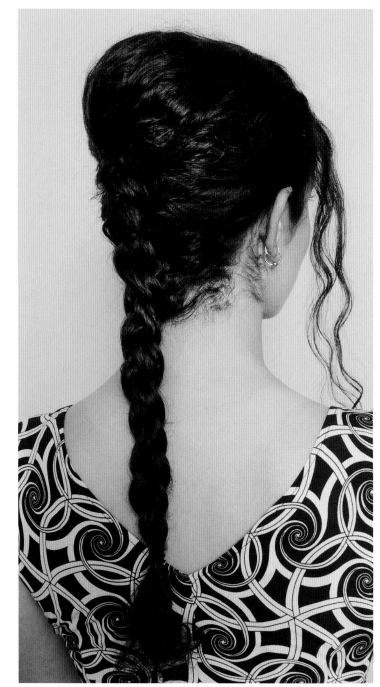

HOW TO DO IT

WHAT YOU NEED

- Comb
- Bobby pins
- Hair tie

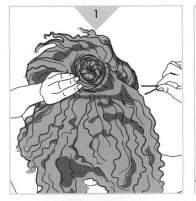

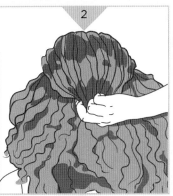

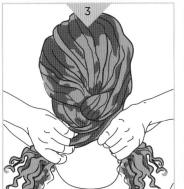

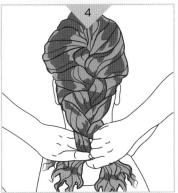

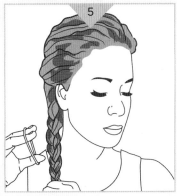

1. Grab a small section of hair, right on top of your head. Twist and wrap this hair into a bun and secure it with bobby pins.

2. Take the hair that sits to the front and sides of the bun, and draw it over the top of the bun to create the illusion of a raised crown. Secure the hair in place with bobby pins.

3. Once the lifted crown is secure, divide your hair into three equal strands to begin your French braid. Include the hair emerging from the raised crown, taking care not to dislodge the pins. Begin French braiding down the center of your head (see page 143 for instructions).

4. Keep braiding and incorporating hair until you reach the nape of your neck, then continue through to the ends.

5. Secure the finished braid with a hair tie.

TOP TIP

If there are visible parts on either side of your head where you have incorporated sections of hair, try smoothing the hair gently with a comb and sliding bobby pins underneath the braid to hold them in position.

MINI SIDE TWISTS

BEST FOR
All hair lengths

ACCESSORIES
Stud this hairstyle with some fancy bobby pins to highlight the twists.

DIFFICULTY LEVEL
Easy

ASSISTANCE NEEDED?
No

I love using twists. They're a great way to show off your curls, and a very easy style to reach for when you're pressed for time. This variation takes only a few minutes once you know what you're doing, and it results in a really cute look. Choose which side of your hair you'd prefer for the placement and have fun!

TRY THIS
As with the other more casual looks in this book, mascara and a bright, fun lip color are all you'll need to make the most of these twists.

SEE ALSO
Triple crown twists, pages 138–39
Half twists, pages 140–41

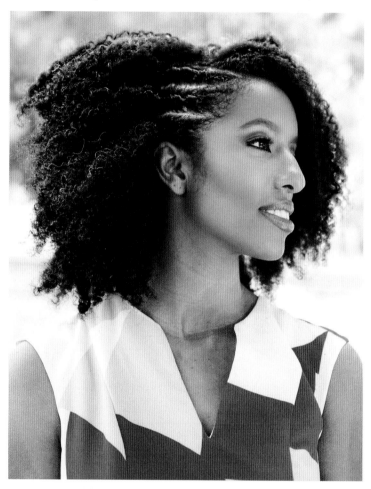

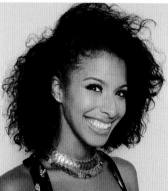

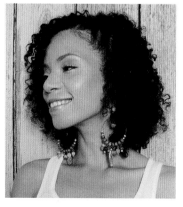

HOW TO DO IT

WHAT YOU NEED

- Comb
- Hair tie
- Bobby pins

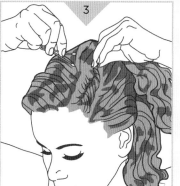
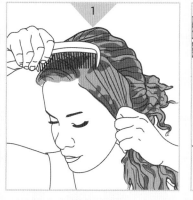
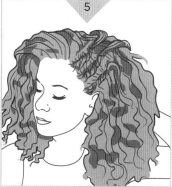
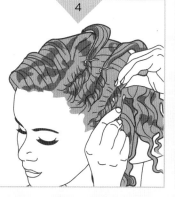
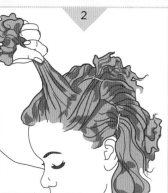

1. Using a comb, make a part slightly to one side of center and separate out a square section running from here down to the front of your ear. Reserve this for your twists and tie the rest of your hair out of the way for now.

2. Divide the square section into three equal subsections, one for each twist. Secure the lower two with hair ties. Take the top subsection in your fingers and, starting at the hairline, twist it until you reach the back of the section.

3. When the twist is complete, slide some bobby pins underneath it to hold it in place.

4. Now repeat the same process with the other two subsections.

5. Finally, release the rest of your hair and puff it out so that it covers the pins while leaving the twists themselves fully visible.

TOP TIP

If your curls are looking a bit lifeless, flip your head over so that your hair falls forward, then massage your curls at the roots to wake them up a bit.

ACCENT BRAIDS

BEST FOR
All hair lengths

ACCESSORIES
Play up the bohemian vibe of this style with dangly earrings.

DIFFICULTY LEVEL
Easy

ASSISTANCE NEEDED?
No

Accent braids are a quick and effective way to jazz up almost any style. The tutorial here features just one small braid on either side, but you are not limited to this—toss in as many braids as you want to make this look your own. The placement of the braids is also up to you. Braids offer one of the easiest ways to be creative, and they always add a festive touch to curly hair.

TRY THIS
These braids provide plenty of texture and interest, so keep your makeup soft and natural. You can let your braids hang alongside your curls, or pin them up to form a hair decoration.

SEE ALSO
Double side braids, pages 144–45
Crown braids, pages 156–57

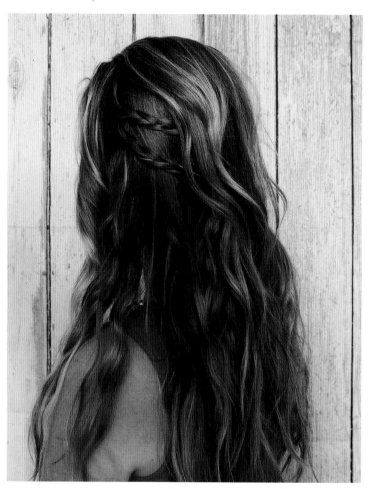

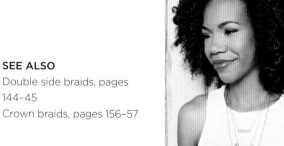

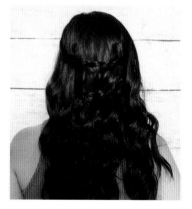

HOW TO DO IT

WHAT YOU NEED

- Hair ties
- Hairspray

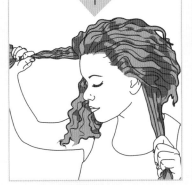

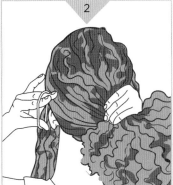

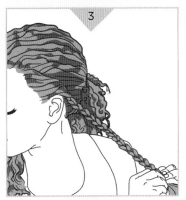

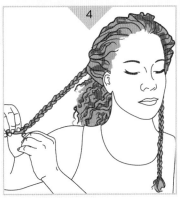

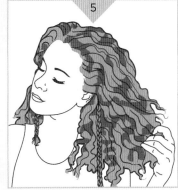

1. The braids in this tutorial will be created just behind the ears, so take a small section of hair on each side at this point. For symmetry, make sure the sections are the same size. (You can, of course, choose to place accent braids anywhere you like!)

2. Leave the small sections sitting forward over your shoulders and tie the rest of your hair out of the way.

3. Braid the first section of hair, working all the way to the very ends, then secure the braid with a hair tie.

4. Do the same with the section on the opposite side.

5. Now release the rest of your hair and plump it up so that it flows freely around the braids. Mist the style with hairspray to fix it in place.

TOP TIP

Small, clear hair ties are great if you can get hold of them—the ends of your braids will then blend more seamlessly into your curls.

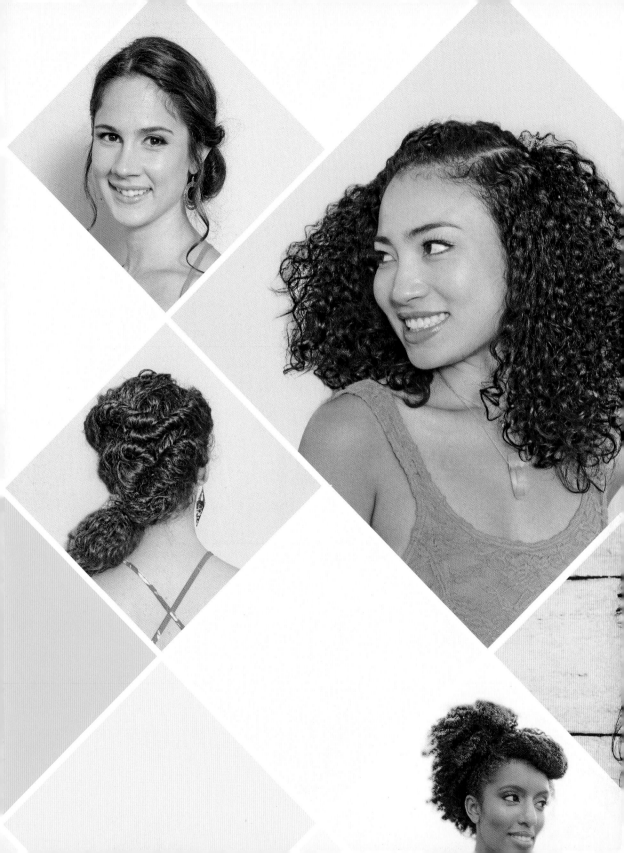

RESOURCES

SCHOOLS AND FURTHER EDUCATION

If you love hair, fashion, and style you might want to look into a career as a cosmetologist.

Hairdressing is a rewarding career that combines technical skills with a creative, communicative outlet, and offers flexibility and the opportunity to run your own freelance business or salon. You'll also be able find work almost anywhere in the world.

Hairdressing is very social, so you will need to be a good communicator and you must be able to keep up with all of your clients' lives. When people go to the salon, it's not just their hair that's expecting attention; people go for an experience.

It's important you understand color, shape, and style, and being able to visualize the end result is vital. Styling hair also takes an impressive number of skills in order to become proficient. Everyone's hair is different, so you'll need to be artistic and creative, with a flair for solving problems. On top of this you'll need to be interested in—and good at—following trends, and be prepared to start your own.

The licensing requirements for cosmetologists and hairdressers vary by state and country, so look for a school in your local area. Below are some helpful links:

North America
Arrojo Cosmetology School (NEW YORK)
arrojocosmetology.com

Aveda Institute (NATIONWIDE AND IN CANADA AND AUSTRALIA)
aveda.edu

Curly Hair Artistry (NORTH CAROLINA)
curlyhairartistry.com

Empire Beauty Schools (NATIONWIDE)
empire.edu

Paul Mitchell Schools (NATIONWIDE)
paulmitchell.edu

Regency Beauty Schools (NATIONWIDE)
regencybeauty.com

BLOGS AND WEBSITES FOR CURLY HAIR TIPS

There are lots of blogs and sites with advice on caring for and working with curly hair. Here are a few:

- ahfrobaang.com (of course!)
- blackgirllonghair.com
- curlynikki.com
- devacurl.com
- hairromance.com
- curlsandblossoms.blogspot.com
- justcurly.com
- mynaturalhairsistas.com
- naturallycurly.com
- thebeautydepartment.com
- themandyexpedition.co.za

OTHER BOOKS IN OUR SERIES

- *Braids, Buns, and Twists!* by Christina Butcher
- *100 Perfect Hair Days* by Jenny Strebe

RIGHT: Half twists, page 140

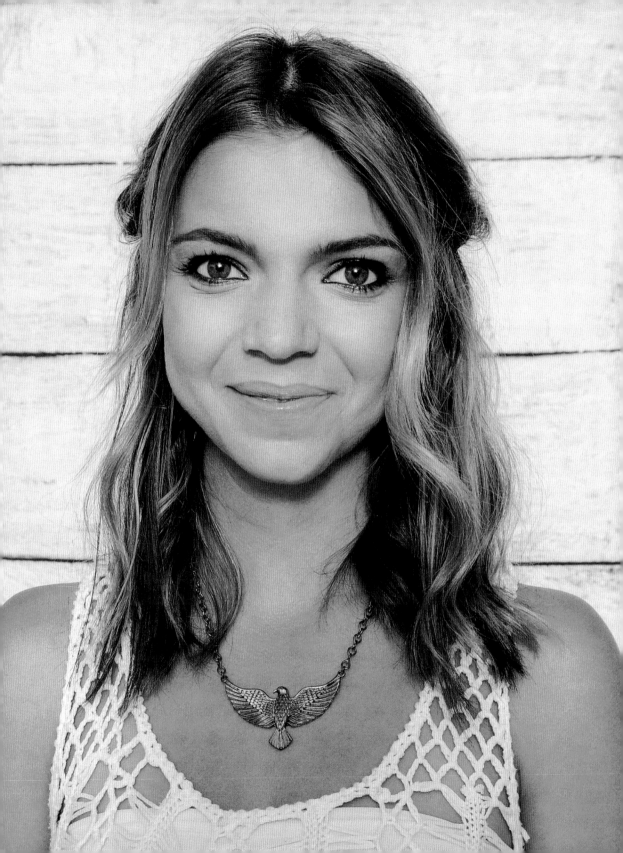

SUPPLIERS

RECOMMENDED BRANDS FOR CURLY HAIR

As I've said elsewhere in this book, the products you choose are a matter of personal choice—you will have the best idea of what works for you. However, experimenting with different brands, and getting advice from friends and professionals, is a great way to discover new favorites, so here are some suggestions. Some of these are U.S. brands, while others come from elsewhere around the world, but many are available internationally, online, or via local stockists.

Afro Deity
afrodeity.co.uk

ApHogee
aphogee.com

As I Am Naturally
asiamnaturally.com

Aunt Jackie's
auntjackiescurlsandcoils.com

Aussie
aussie.com

Aveda
aveda.com

BeUnique Hair Care
beuniquehaircare.co.uk

Big Hair Beauty
bighair.co.uk

Boots Essentials
boots.com

Bumble and Bumble
bumbleandbumble.com

Camille Rose Naturals
camillerosenaturals.com

Carol's Daughter
carolsdaughter.com

Coco Curls
naturallycurly.com

Creme Of Nature
cremeofnature.com

Curl Junkie
curljunkie.com

Curls
curlsbiz.com

Curly by Nature
curlybynature.com

Curly Ellie
curlyellie.com

Dark and Lovely
worldwide stockists

Design Essentials
designessentials.com

Deva Curl
devacurl.com

Dr. Organic
drorganic.co.uk

EDEN BodyWorks
eden-bodyworks.myshopify.com

Elucence
elucence.com

Jane Carter Solution
janecartersolution.com

Jessicurl
jessicurl.com

Kinky-Curly
kinky-curly.com

Lotta Body
lottabody.com

Lush
lushusa.com

Mahogany Naturals
mahoganynaturals.co.uk

Mane Divas
manedivas.co.uk

Mixed Chicks
mixedchicks.net

Mizani
mizani.com

Ouidad
ouidad.com

Oyin Handmade
oyinhandmade.com

Shea Moisture
sheamoisture.com

SheaButter Cottage
sheabuttercottage.com

Superdrug
superdrug.com

Thank God It's Natural
thankgodimnatural.com

TIGI
worldwide stockists

Vatika Naturals
vatikanaturals.co.uk

Wen
wenhaircair.ca

RECOMMENDED TOOLS

A few more recommendations. All of these are available online, via the manufacturers or third-party stockists.

Aquis hair towels

Boucleme curl towel

Curlformers

Curly Hair Solutions bonnet hood dryer

Denman brushes

DevaCurl "Deva Towel"

Diane Twist-Flex Rods

Hair Therapy thermal turban heat wrap

Hot Sock ultralight diffuser

"No Snag" soft hair bands

NuBone II Finish Pro detangler

Q-Redew steamer

SLAPS satin-lined caps

Spilo duckbill clips

GLOSSARY

Backcombing

Also known as teasing, rattling, matting, or French lacing. This technique involves combing small sections of hair toward the scalp, creating an underlying cushion or base for hairstyles that need volume.

Bangs

Also known as a fringe, this is the front section of hair that falls across the forehead. You can style bangs in lots of ways, and they can be long or short, straight or curved, wispy or full; they can also be parted, sideswept, or straight down. You can opt to leave bangs loose, or include them in your chosen hairstyle.

Bobby pins

The simplest kind of hair pin. Usually metal, about two inches long and with one straight prong pressed against a slightly wavier one to grip the hair.

Braiding

A styling technique that involves weaving three strands of hair into each other. There are several ways you can braid your hair including simple three-strand braids, Dutch braids, and French braids.

Cornrow

A form of braid woven tight against the scalp and incorporating surrounding hair along its length, like a Dutch braid but much smaller.

Co-wash

Using conditioner instead of shampoo to wash the hair, a technique that allows the hair to retain its natural oils.

Crown

The upper back of the head, surrounding the high crown.

Curl definer

A styling lotion that helps to control frizz, add moisture, and give curls a definite yet manageable hold. Can be used on wet or dry hair.

Dutch braid

A braiding technique that crosses sections of hair under one another, while drawing new hair in from either side of the braid in turn. This is essentially an inverted French braid, where the resulting braid sits on top of the hair, rather than below it.

Fishtail braid

A technique that takes two even strands and interweaves them, crisscrossing a small strand from each side back over the other in alternate steps, to create a thick and densely woven braid with the appearance of two interconnected strands.

French braid

A braiding technique that crosses sections of hair over one another, while also drawing new hair in from either side of the braid. The French braid has a flatter appearance than its Dutch cousin due to the movement of the strands passing over and down rather than under and up at each step.

Hair clip

A long, slim clip used for holding sections of hair out of the way during styling.

Hair donut

A fat, round hairband that can be used to style your hair into a distinctive bun and provide extra fullness to thinner hair.

Hair extensions

Additional hair that is attached to your natural hair to add length, volume, or texture. Extensions can be permanently attached with glue or tape, or temporarily clipped in.

Hair pick

A comb with long, wide teeth, which can be made of metal or of plastic.

Hair texture

A term used to classify hair type, depending on the curl pattern, volume, and consistency of the hair.

Hair tie

Also known as a hair elastic.
A small, stretchy ring used to tie
and hold hair in place.

Hairline

The line that stretches along
the edges of the area where
your hair naturally grows,
including around your face,
ears, and neckline.

High crown

The highest point of the crown
on the back of the head.

Microfiber towel

A high-tech towel with an
amazing ability to soak up water.
These will save you on drying
time and are much gentler than
an ordinary towel.

Mousse

A light, fast-drying foam that
gives extra volume, texture, and
shine. It can be used on wet or
dry hair.

Nape

The back of the neck, below the
natural hairline.

Neck

A term for the part of a person's
body that connects the head to
the rest of the body.

Protein treatment

An intensive treatment used
to build strength and a smooth
texture back into hair. Protein
treatments can be commercially

produced or homemade using
natural ingredients, and are
sometimes set using heat
after application.

Serum

A hair product used to control
frizz, smooth flyaways and
strays, and add shine.

Sulfate-free shampoo

Shampoo that is free from
sulfates and other chemicals
that can dry out your hair.

Teasing

See backcombing.

CONTRIBUTORS AND CREDITS

All location photography

Yolanda Diaz
(executive)
yolandadiaz.us

Blogger photographs

Genevieve Jauquet, 132, 166

Other images
Getty Images, 16–20

Hairstylists

Samantha Harris
(executive)

Hannah Erickson

Genevieve Jauquet

Lauren Jauquet

Stylists

Samantha Harris

Hannah Erickson

Crystal Harris

Makeup artists

Samantha Harris

Genevieve Jauquet

Models

Rose Marie Balistrieri, 8, 10, 43
110, 152

Nicole Baulknight, 11, 39, 53, 82,
94, 96, 166, 178

Fernanda Chamorro, 6, 10, 15, 52,
54, 60, 64, 76, 142, 146, 148, 158,
168, 176

Cage Cluff, 8, 11, 15, 31, 66, 86,
92, 104, 150, 154, 158, 162, 164,
168, 172

Maureen Eppler, 11, 72, 158

Hannah Erickson, 7–8, 10, 15, 78,
82, 90, 94–95, 100, 108, 112, 124,
128, 133, 140, 152, 179, 181

Alanna Evans, 6–8, 11, 22, 52,
56, 80, 88, 95–96, 102, 112, 132,
156, 170

Clarissa Evans, 7, 14, 74, 78, 112,
120, 126, 138, 144, 152, 162, 191

Crystal Harris, 136, 174

Samantha Harris, 5, 6–9, 13, 42,
60, 66, 68, 74, 84, 102, 114, 116,
118, 128

Marissa Henson, 9–10 86, 104,
130, 132, 156

Aly Hill, 4, 6–7, 9, 11, 15, 27, 42, 52,
68, 86, 94, 98, 110, 116, 120, 124,
140, 174

Rachel Jordan, 4, 9, 11, 68, 90,
100, 116, 120, 122, 133, 164, 174, 178

Esther Marie, 5–8, 10, 32, 42–43,
53, 72, 76, 82, 88, 95, 98, 100,
142, 146, 150, 154

Illayda Rosier, 6, 9–11, 36, 42–43,
58, 62, 126, 132, 134, 148, 154, 162,
168, 178–79, 187

Victoria Louise Scott, 7–10, 14,
80, 98, 110, 114, 124, 126, 133,
138, 179

Bethany Shedrick, 8–9, 14, 35,
62, 66, 74, 84, 90, 102, 106, 108,
114, 122, 136, 144, 156, 160, 170

Christina Smith, 56, 88

Tiffany Marie Stephens, 6, 10–11,
14, 43, 52–54, 58, 64, 70, 94–95,
104, 108, 133, 144,
148, 176

RIGHT: Cinammon roll
braid, page 162

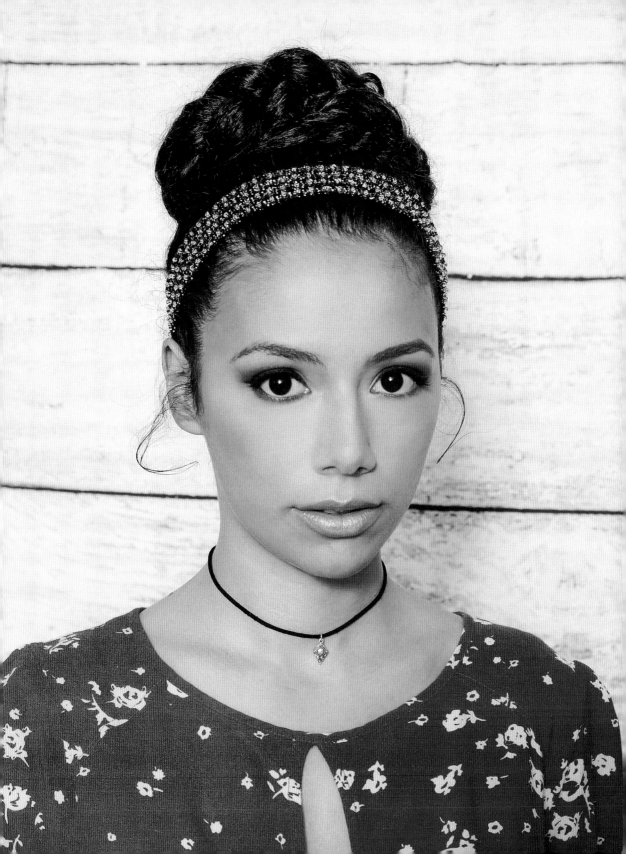

INDEX

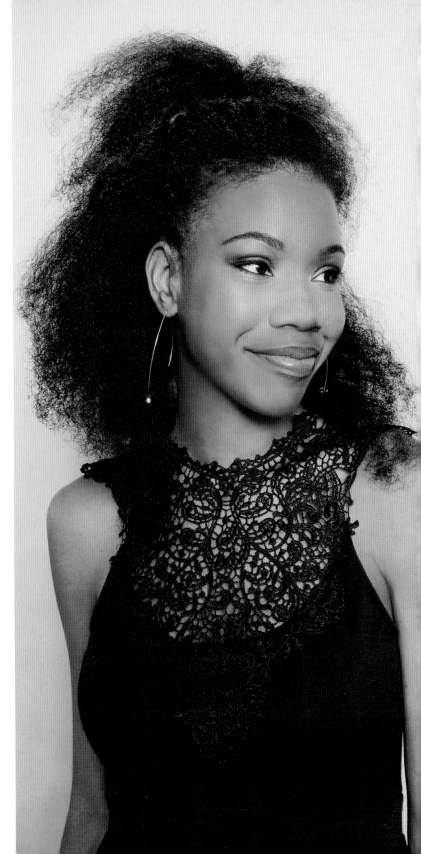

RIGHT: Twisted half-up ponytail, page 78

ACKNOWLEDGMENTS

This book has been a wonderful experience and would not have been possible without the help of some key people in my life who inspired me along the way. Thank you to Andrew Schmitt, who consistently encouraged me throughout the entire journey, pre-editing my writing, taking my step-by-step photos for the illustrator, and helping me at each photo shoot. You have been nothing short of a miracle and I am very blessed to have you in my life.

To my sisters, Vicky and Christie, who encourage and inspire me to be a better person every day. My nephews and nieces, Joshua, Jordan, Faith, and Journey, who help me to see the world with bright eyes. Thank you. To my hairstylist and business partner, Hannah Erickson, who pushed past her limits at every photo shoot and re-created some amazing hairstyles. Thank you for teaching me how to style better and for opening up your schedule to do this project with me. To my amazing photographer Yolanda Diaz, who is so great at what she does—thank you for all the hours of hosting, shooting, and editing the photos for this project.

Genevieve Jauquet, thank you for contributing to this project with your hair and makeup skills, and for pepping me up with positivity along the way. To Jai Hayes and Melanie Allen, who have helped me perfect my writing skills and encouraged me to step outside of my comfort zone.

To Isheeta Mustafi, Abbie Sharman, and Angela Koo for consistently pushing me to excel and believing in me. Thank you for hanging in there with me and being so supportive.

To all of the models and bloggers who made time to be a part of this project, thank you. Finally, to all of my online family and any and everyone in my life who has been in my corner. I am forever grateful to you.